Transdermal Delivery of Drugs

Volume III

Editors

Agis F. Kydonieus, Ph.D.
President
Hercon Laboratories Corporation
Subsidiary of Health-Chem Corporation
South Plainfield, New Jersey

Bret Berner, Ph.D.
Manager
Pharmaceutical Division
Ciba-Geigy Corporation
Ardsley, New York

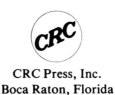

CRC Press, Inc.
Boca Raton, Florida

Library of Congress Cataloging-in-Publication Data

Transdermal delivery of drugs.

   Includes bibliographies and index.
   1. Ointments. 2. Skin absorption. 3. Drugs--
Controlled release. I. Kydonieus, Agis F., 1938-
II. Berner, Bret. [DNLM: 1. Administration, Topical.
2. Delayed-Action Preparations. 3. Drugs--administra-
tion & dosage. 4. Skin Absorption. WB 340 T7723]
RS201.03T7255   1987   615'.67   86-2585
ISBN 0-8493-6483-3 (set)
ISBN 0-8493-6484-1 (v. 1)
ISBN 0-8493-6485-X (v. 2)
ISBN 0-8493-6486-8 (v. 3)

Direct all inquiries to CRC Press, Inc., 2000 Corporate Blvd., N.W., Boca Raton, Florida, 33431.

International Standard Book Number 0-8493-6483-3 (set)
International Standard Book Number 0-8493-6484-1 (v. 1)
International Standard Book Number 0-8493-6485-X (v. 2)
International Standard Book Number 0-8493-6486-8 (v. 3)

Library of Congress Card Number 86-2585
Printed in the United States

PREFACE

The introduction of the first transdermal patch containing scopolamine brought about a tremendous interest in the usage of intact skin as a portal of entry of drugs into the systemic circulation of the body. Several transdermal products followed into the marketplace, in particular, devices containing nitroglycerin, clonidine, isosorbide dinitrate (Japan), and estradiol (Switzerland). Some two dozen drugs are now in different steps of transdermal product development. A plethora of transdermal development departments and companies have emerged. While the potential advantages of transdermal delivery such as (1) avoidance of hepatic ''first-pass'' metabolism, (2) maintenance of steady-state plasma levels of drug, and (3) convenience of dosing were readily identified, the limitations of the barrier and immune properties of skin are only now being defined. Continued technological advances are requiring either circumventing these responses of the skin or adroit identification of conditions in search of controlled-release therapies. The goals of these volumes are to collect the current knowledge to further research in transdermal delivery and to serve as an introduction to the novice.

The series of volumes is divided into four main sections pertaining to Methodology, The Transdermal Device, The Skin, and The Drug. For the recent practitioner in the field, an overview section has been included to provide a background about the controlled release devices, the diffusion of drugs through polymers, and the anatomy and biochemistry of skin.

In the methodology section, the techniques used to determine in vitro and in vivo skin permeation are presented. The special considerations concerning animal and human experimentation are described including in vivo methodology, skin condition, and individual variations.

A section on transdermal devices concludes the first volume. Here we asked scientists from six companies to discuss briefly their transdermal technology and product development areas.

The volume on skin contains chapters on the parameters affecting skin penetration, including a chapter on aging, pharmacokinetics of transdermal delivery, models for predicting the permeability of drugs through skin from the physicochemical parameters of the drug, the correlations among human skin, reconstituted skin, artificial membranes, and the potential of increasing skin permeability by the use of chemical enhancers or vehicles. Finally, a chapter on the crucial area of cutaneous toxicology describes contact dermatitis and microorganism growth and infections.

In the third volume, the drug parameters important to transdermal delivery are discussed. The thermodynamics governing transdermal delivery and models and typical approaches for prodrugs are also presented. Finally, a literature review of the permeability of drugs through the skin is presented. This compilation of existing skin permeation data should serve as a useful reference tool.

Obviously, in this rapidly expanding field, several important omissions must have occurred despite our effort to include significant developments known by 1984, when most of the manuscripts were collected. Nevertheless, we hope this effort will prove to be of value to scientists and product development engineers seeking up-to-date information in this area.

We are indebted to the authors for their cooperation in adhering to manuscript specifications and to Mrs. Robin Tyminski for her efforts in typing and assisting in the editorial endeavors. Finally, we would like to thank the management of Health-Chem Corporation, the parent of Hercon Laboratories, who have been strong advocates of controlled release for many years and have given the editors all the support required to complete this undertaking.

Agis F. Kydonieus
Bret Berner

THE EDITORS

Agis F. Kydonieus, Ph.D., is President of Hercon Laboratories Corporation, a subsidiary of Health-Chem Corporation, New York. Dr. Kydonieus graduated from the University of Florida in 1959 with a B.S. degree in Chemical Engineering (summa cum laude) and received his Ph.D. from the same school in 1964.

Dr. Kydonieus is a founder of the Controlled Release Society and has served as a member of the Board of Governors, Program Chairman, Vice President, and President. He is presently a trustee of the Society. He is also founder of Krikos, an international Hellenic association of scientists, and has served a treasurer and a member of its Board of Directors. He is also a member of the editorial board of the *Journal of Controlled Release,* and a member of many societies including the American Association of Pharmaceutical Scientists, American Institute of Chemical Engineers, and the Society of Plastics Engineers.

Dr. Kydonieus is the author of over 125 patents, publications, and presentations in the field of controlled release and biomedical devices. He is the Editor of *Controlled Release Technologies* and *Insect Suppression with Controlled Release Pheromone Systems,* both published with CRC Press.

Bret Berner, Ph.D., is Manager of Basic Pharmaceutics Research for CIBA-GEIGY, Inc. Dr. Berner received his B.A. degree from the University of Rochester in 1973 and his Ph.D. from the University of California at Los Angeles in 1978. Before joining CIBA-GEIGY in 1985, he was Director of Research, Hercon Division of Health-Chem Corporation. Dr. Berner also held the position of staff scientist with Proctor & Gamble, Co. following his graduation from UCLA.

Dr. Berner's current research directs novel drug delivery research groups including transdermal, gastrointestinal, and other delivery routes, polymer systems, pharmacokinetics, pharmacodynamics, and analytical chemistry.

CONTRIBUTORS

Joseph J. Anisko, Ph.D.
Director of Information and
  Communications
Nelson Research and Development
Irvine, California

Charanjit R. Behl
Pharmaceutical Research and
  Development
Hoffmann-La Roche, Inc.
Nutley, New Jersey

Nancy H. Bellantone
Pharmaceutical Research
Pfizer, Inc.
Groton, Connecticut

Bret Berner, Ph.D.
Manager
Pharmaceutical Division
Ciba-Geigy Corp.
Ardsley, New York

S. Kumar Chandrasekaran
Vice President, Technical Affairs
Sola-Syntex Ophthalmics
Phoenix, Arizona

Eugene R. Cooper, Ph.D.
Alcon Labs, Inc.
Fort Worth, Texas

Gordon L. Flynn, Ph.D.
Professor
Department of Pharmaceuticals
College of Pharmacy
University of Michigan
Ann Arbor, Michigan

Sharad K. Govil
Research and Development
Key Pharmaceuticals, Inc.
Pembroke Pines, Florida

Gary Lee Grove, Ph.D.
Director
Skin Study Center
Philadelphia, Pennsylvania

Richard H. Guy, Ph.D.
Assistant Professor of Pharmacy and
  Pharmaceutical Chemistry
Departments of Pharmacy and
  Pharmaceutical Chemistry
University of California
San Francisco, California

Jonathan Hadgraft, D.phil.
Professor of Pharmaceutical Chemistry
The Welsh School of Pharmacy
University of Wales Institute of Science
  and Technology
Cardiff, Wales, U.K.

Timothy A. Hagan
College of Pharmacy
University of Michigan
Ann Arbor, Michigan

W.I. Higuchi, Ph.D.
Distinguished Professor and Chairman
Department of Pharmaceutics
College of Pharmacy
University of Utah
Salt Lake City, Utah

Sui Yuen E. Hou
College of Pharmacy
University of Michigan
Ann Arbor, Michigan

Bernard Idson, Ph.D.
Senior Research Fellow
Department of Pharmacy Research and
  Development
Hoffmann-La Roche, Inc.
Nutley, New Jersey

Benjamin K. Kim
Director, Drug Delivery Systems
Nelson Research
Irvine, California

Tamie Kurihara-Bergstrom
Ciba-Geigy Corp.
Ardsley, New York

Agis F. Kydonieus, Ph.D.
Executive Vice President
Hercon Division
Health-Chem Corp.
South Plainfield, New Jersey

James J. Leyden, M.D.
Professor of Dermatology
Department of Dermatology
University of Pennsylvania
Philadelphia, Pennsylvania

Edward E. Linn
Formulations Research
Lederle Labs
American Cyanamid
Pearl River, New York

Vithal Rajadhyaksha
Sr. Vice President Research and
  Development
Nelson Research Centerpointe
Irvine, California

Pramod P. Sarpotdar, Ph.D.
Senior Research Scientist
Research Laboratories
Eastman Kodak Co.
Rochester, New York

Ward M. Smith
College of Pharmacy
University of Michigan
Ann Arbor, Michigan

Rajaram Vaidyanathan, Ph.D.
Director
Product Development
Nelson Research
Irvine, California

David Yeung, M.S.
Senior Research Investigator
Dermatological Research
Richardson-Vicks Incorporated
Shelton, Connecticut

Cheng-Der Yu
Manager
Pharmaceutical Development
Cooper Laboratories, Inc.
Mountain View, California

Joel L. Zatz. Ph.D.
Professor of Pharmaceutics
College of Pharmacy
Rutgers College of Pharmacy
Piscataway, New Jersey

TABLE OF CONTENTS

Volume II

SKIN

Volume III

DRUG

Drug

Chapter 1

DRUG PARAMETERS IMPORTANT FOR TRANSDERMAL DELIVERY

Richard H. Guy and Jonathan Hadgraft

TABLE OF CONTENTS

I. INTRODUCTION

Transdermal drug delivery to achieve systemic pharmacological effect is now recognized as a viable means to administer therapeutic agents. Devices have been described for the delivery of such diverse molecules as scopolamine,[1] nitroglycerin,[2-4] clonidine,[5] and estradiol.[6] However, the range of chemical types encompassed by these drugs should not lead one to assume that transdermal delivery will be successful for all species. Indeed, there are important limitations upon the properties of the agent to be delivered such that many drugs in common use are precluded from this mode of administration. It is the purpose of this chapter to identify the drug criteria which determine the feasibility of transdermal delivery. We have chosen to consider the relevant drug parameters in three categories:

1.   Biological
2.   Physicochemical
3.   Pharmacokinetic

We shall address each of these in turn and conclude by providing examples for which the various contributory factors come together to predict the possible success of the transdermal delivery route.

II. BIOLOGICAL CRITERIA

A. Therapeutic Index (TI)

With respect to the TI of the drug, the classic controlled delivery figure (Figure 1) encapsulates the required criteria for transdermal input. Administration must lead to plasma levels (or, more specifically, drug concentrations in the "biophase") above the minimum effective concentration (MEC) but below the minimum toxic concentration (MTC). The sustained delivery should produce steady levels of circulating drug and overcome, thereby, the "sawtooth" profile produced by more conventional dosing regimens, e.g., multiple oral doses. In this way, one may maintain the drug concentration within the TI, minimize the occurrence of side effects, and improve patient compliance.

As we shall see, however, for transdermal drug delivery, the therapeutic agent must be potent if the administration route is to be a feasible option. To date, the excellent barrier properties of the stratum corneum have limited the drugs chosen for transdermal delivery to those whose daily dose requirements are on the order of mg/day. In the majority of cases, this translates into a plasma concentration of approximately ng/mℓ. It remains to be seen whether, with the use of penetration enhancers, for example, the biophase level of active agent can be increased further without resorting to an unacceptable surface area of contact between skin and device. More discussion and illustration of these points is presented later in this chapter.

B. Drug Inactivation

A frequently cited advantage of transdermal input is the ability to avoid inactivation of the drug through a hepatic first-pass effect or by GI degradation. This observation is perhaps best exemplified by nitroglycerin (NTG) which is not only subject to major metabolic clearance by the liver but is also decomposed by circulating red blood cells.[7,8]

C. Biological Half-Life (t$_{1/2}$)

The t$_{1/2}$ criterion for drugs administered transcutaneously is that which characterizes all forms of sustained or prolonged delivery; namely, that the half-life be short rather than long. If the t$_{1/2}$ is large then, because percutaneous absorption is, on the whole, a slow process,

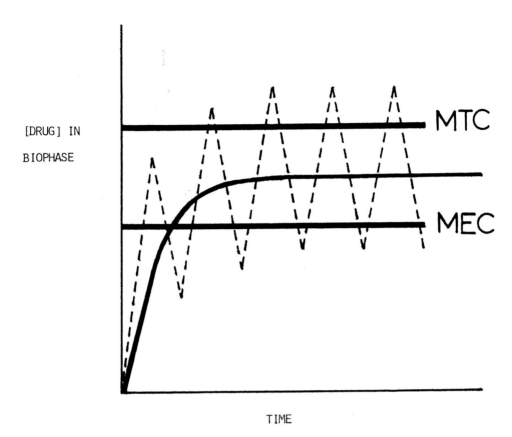

TIME

FIGURE 1.   The classic goal of controlled drug input: the rapid attainment of a steady prolonged biophase level within the therapeutic index. The profile is contrasted with that resulting from multiple doses of a "conventional" formulation (leading to the "sawtooth" pattern and periods of both over- and underdosing).

the attainment of steady-state plasma levels will be delayed considerably. We may illustrate this point using in vivo transdermal delivery data for NTG and clonidine.[9,10] Plasma levels following administration of these two drugs to human volunteers are shown in Figure 2. In both studies, the results of which are combined on this figure, drug was delivered from a "membrane-controlled" patch of similar design. It is immediately apparent that steady-state levels of NTG ($t_{1/2} \simeq 2$ min[11]) are achieved much more rapidly than those of clonidine ($t_{1/2} \simeq 10$ hr[11]). Although there are physicochemical factors which also influence the time to steady state in these situations, none is capable of exerting such a dramatic effect as the $t_{1/2}$.

D. Limiting Factors
Finally, in this section, it is appropriate to highlight three potential biological limitations to transdermal drug delivery.

1.   The administered drug must not induce a cutaneous irritant or allergic response.
2.   Because the barrier nature of skin ensures that transdermal input provides rather constant delivery of drug, it is important that the pharmacological effect of the agent be suited to this absorption behavior. In other words, one must be careful to ascertain that tolerance to the drug does not develop under the near zero-order profile of transdermal delivery.
3.   Cutaneous metabolism remains an essentially unknown variable in topical drug delivery. The skin does contain multiple enzyme systems many of which are capable of

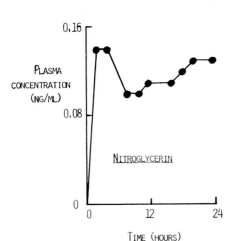
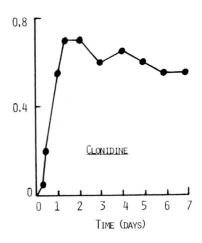

FIGURE 2.   In vivo plasma concentration vs. time data for NTG and clonidine following transdermal delivery.[9,10] The difference in rates of attainment of steady-state blood levels reflects primarily the difference in the biological half-lives of the two drugs.

converting transporting drug molecules to metabolite species.[12] Thus, the possibility of a significant cutaneous first-pass effect exists. Experimental determinations of the simultaneous transport and bioconversion of penetrating molecules are sparse and inconclusive as to the potential importance of cutaneous metabolism; in particular, unambiguous in vivo demonstration of the phenomenon is difficult. With respect to transdermal drug delivery, a recent study of NTG absorption in rhesus monkeys[13] offers the most relevant evidence. In this investigation, it was concluded that a skin first-pass effect of 15 to 20% could be inferred from the results. If such an effect proves to be more generally true, then we may expect a considerable amount of activity in this research area during the next few years. Elsewhere, in connection with topical drug administration, in vitro studies have shown that excised skin remains enzymatically viable.[14-16] The possible ramifications of these observations have also been subjected to theoretical treatment;[17-20] the implications of this work are considerable and await experimental test. Parenthetically, one should add that bacteria are present on the skin surface and that these microflora are possible inactivators of transdermally delivered drugs. The occlusive environment beneath a therapeutic system may present an attractive region for this interaction.

III. PHYSICOCHEMICAL CRITERIA

In asking the question, "what physicochemical criteria determine the feasibility of delivering a drug transdermally", it is instructive to identify the sequential physical processes which a drug, presented in a topical delivery system, must undergo to become available in the systemic circulation. These events may be summarized as follows:

1.   Drug transport within the delivery system to the device-skin surface interface
2.   Partitioning of drug from the delivery system into the stratum corneum
3.   Diffusion of drug across the stratum corneum
4.   Drug partitioning from the stratum corneum into the viable epidermis.
5.   Transport of drug through the viable tissue
6.   Drug uptake by the cutaneous microcapillary network and subsequent systemic distribution.

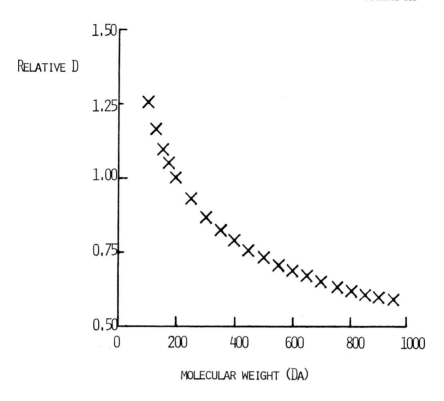

FIGURE 3.   Idealized dependence of solute diffusion coefficient (D) upon molecular weight (M) according to Equation 1. The ordinate expresses a relative D, normalized with respect to that of a molecule of molecular weight 200 daltons.

The key words, which are pertinent to this stage of the discussion, therefore, are diffusion and partitioning.

A. Diffusion

The transport characteristics of the drug are determined primarily by its size and by its level of interaction with the media through which diffusion is taking place, i.e., delivery system, stratum corneum, viable epidermis. Most drugs in current use have molecular weights of less than 1000 daltons. Beyond this magnitude, organic molecules tend to fall into categories such as polymers or peptides, for which, we shall see, there are overriding factors that control penetration. For the smaller species (< 1000 daltons), the effect of size on diffusion in liquids may be viewed in terms of the Stokes-Einstein equation, that is

$$D = C \cdot M^{-1/3} \qquad (1)$$

where M is molecular weight and C is a constant. Although this is an ideal equation which makes the assumption that the molecules are spherical, it does provide a reasonable estimate of the size effect on diffusion. It also implies that the molecular weight plays a rather minor role in influencing D, i.e., the $M^{-1/3}$ function is not very powerful; see Figure 3.

However, it is clear from the literature[21] that the diffusion coefficient of chemicals through the skin, e.g., the stratum corneum, is very sensitive to the nature of the penetrant, in specific to the degree of interaction between the molecule and the tissue. Scheuplein and Blank,[22] for example, have quoted values of D (for stratum corneum transport) ranging from 10^{-13} to 10^{-9} cm²/sec. The diffusion coefficients were inferred from permeability data through excised skin and the substances studied encompassed a range which included water,

Table 1
IN VITRO SKIN PERMEABILITY
COEFFICIENTS (P) OF TWO HOMOLOGOUS
GROUPS OF STEROIDS

Steroid	Hydroxyl groups	Carbonyl groups	$10^6 P$/cm/hr
Progesterone	0	2	1500
Hydroxyprogesterone	1	2	600
Cortexone	1	2	450
Cortexolone	2	2	75
Cortisone	2	3	10
Cortisol	3	2	3
Estrone	1	1	3600
Estradiol	2	0	300
Estriol	3	0	40

simple alcohols, and a number of steroids. The evaluation of D from the experimental data required the assumption of a specific diffusion path length through the stratum corneum; thus, while the absolute magnitudes of the D values quoted may not be precise, the span of the data, i.e., D varying over four orders of magnitude, is representative. Of course, one must realize that the experimental observation is an *apparent* diffusion coefficient which contains information about the degree of interaction or binding between the penetrant and skin. Seemingly minor changes in chemical structure, therefore, can lead to dramatic alterations in permeation behavior, for example, Scheuplein et al. demonstrated an enormous range of permeability coefficients for a closely related series of steroidal molecules[23] (see Table 1). It seems clear that the introduction of increasing polarity into a molecular backbone leads to significant dimunition in skin penetration capability.

B. Partitioning

Among the six sequential steps in percutaneous absorption identified above, there are two key partitioning processes, between the delivery system and the stratum corneum and between the lipophilic stratum corneum and the much more aqueous in nature viable epidermis.

Hence, the partitioning criteria demanded of a drug candidate for transdermal delivery are severe. First, the molecule must favor the stratum corneum over the device and then, the relative affinity of the drug for stratum corneum and viable tissue must be reasonably balanced (to ensure adequate throughput of material into the systemic circulation). Thus, extreme partitioning characteristics are not conducive to successful drug delivery via the skin.

Although it is inappropriate here to review comprehensively the literature pertaining to drug penetration as a function of partition coefficient, it is instructive to consider a few illustrations of such work. Human skin absorption has been correlated with a heptane-aqueous buffer partition coefficient (K).[24] Agreement was reasonable for the most oil-soluble and the most water-soluble penetrants but the intermediate range of compounds were not differentiated in any consistent fashion. The permeability of human epidermis to phenolic compounds in vitro has been measured.[25] Penetration could be related to the substrate K(octanol/water) provided that the applied concentration of phenol did not damage the cutaneous barrier. Steroid penetration in man has been studied[26] and a reasonable coincidence was found between estimated half-lives for penetration and benzene solubility. A linear free energy relationship between the bioresponse and the physical chemical quantity was calculated. Lien and Tong[27] have also used the extrathermodynamic approach to establish linear

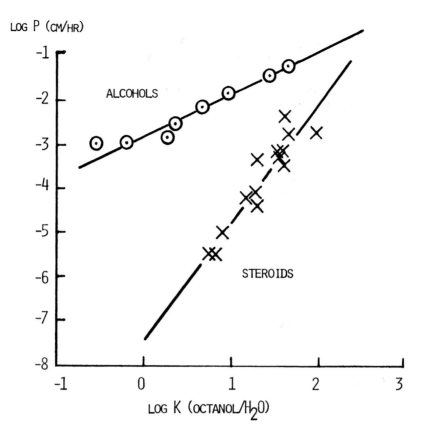

FIGURE 4. Examples of linear relationships between in vitro skin permeability and log K (octanol/water).[27]

equations between penetration and log K(octanol/H$_2$O) (see Figure 4). They concluded that the lipophilic character of the compound, as measured by K, plays the most crucial role in determining skin absorption. Elsewhere, the penetration of the homologous series of *n*-alkanols has been considered.[28,29] Good agreement between K(ether/water) and in vitro permeability was found up to octanol but the behavior of subsequent members of the series indicated that a change of rate-limiting step was occurring when the hydrophobicity reached a certain level. Overall, therefore, one may conclude that there is likely to be some degree of correlation between K and in vivo percutaneous absorption. However, at the present time, K must not be considered predictive, merely indicative of probable high or probable low penetration. Both lipid and water solubility, to some extent, appears necessary for transdermal passage — more specific definition of a relation between a consistent physical parameter (or parameters) and a validated measure of expected permeability in man awaits identification.

Finally, mention should be made of the potential role of the pK of the drug. It is generally agreed that ionized species penetrate the skin considerably less well than their nonionized counterparts. For example, the in vitro permeation of scopolamine from solutions at three different pH values has been reported.[30] The data are summarized in Table 2, which shows clearly how absorption increases as the pH is raised above the pK (7.35) of the weakly basic drug. There is also more recent evidence that the ionization properties of drugs may be used to unexpected advantage.[31] Facilitated transport of salicylate as an ion pair with amine derivatives has been reported in a novel diffusion cell procedure. It is possible, furthermore, that a similar mechanism accounts for the enhanced penetration rate of indomethacin at pH 6.2;[32] support is lent to this hypothesis by the fact that *bis*(2-hydroxypropyl)amine was

Table 2
THE EFFECT OF pH ON THE IN VITRO SKIN FLUX (J) OF SCOPOLAMINE

[Scopolamine] in donor compartment (mg/mℓ)	pH of donor solution	Av J at 30°C (μg/cm²/hr)
520	4.0	1.3
52	4.0	0.13
5.2	4.0	0.016
470	6.6	2.2
47	6.6	0.19
4.7	6.6	0.03
110	9.6	3.6
11	9.6	0.15
1.1	9.6	0.025

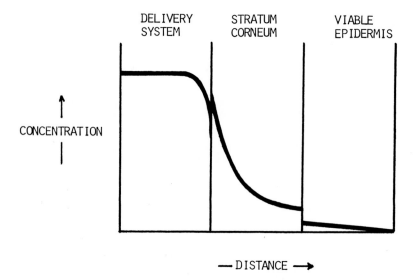

FIGURE 5.   Schematic, nonsteady state, concentration profile applicable to transdermal drug delivery.

present in the topical preparation and because the pK of indomethacin is 5.2. The potential to use facilitated transport in transdermal delivery, therefore, warrants continued consideration.

IV. PHARMACOKINETIC CRITERIA

The rigorous approach for understanding the pharmacokinetics of transdermal drug delivery requires solution of the nonsteady-state diffusion equation (Fick's 2nd law).

$$\partial c/\partial t = D\ \partial^2 c/\partial x^2 \tag{2}$$

for the device, the stratum corneum, and the viable epidermis (see Figure 5). As one might expect, the solutions to these equations are complex and often require that the problem be simplified somewhat so that analytical expressions for amount penetrating per unit time can be obtained.[33-36] The reward for such effort is a direct physicochemical insight into those penetrant properties which have major influence upon the absorption rate. Such an approach is included in another chapter in Volume I.

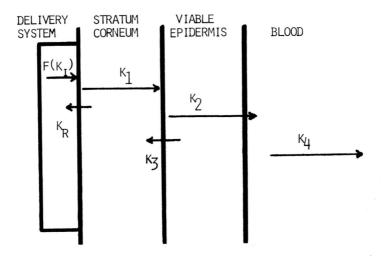

FIGURE 6. A pharmacokinetic model for transdermal drug delivery.[42-44]

However, the utility of this attack on the problem remains theoretical rather than practical and a more pragmatic approach becomes necessary to identify the pharmacokinetic drug criteria which are important in transdermal delivery. Therefore, the use of linear, first-order kinetic models has developed.[37-39] While these simulations can adequately and simply interpret the observed data, they lack the ability to provide any physical meaning to the rate parameters derived.

Most recently, we have attempted to resolve the dilemma by establishing a biophysical pharmacokinetic model for percutaneous absorption in which the rate constants are assigned true physicochemical significance and may be predicted from basic physical properties.[40,41] The extension of this model to include drug input from a transdermal patch is illustrated in Figure 6.[42-44] The kinetic parameters are associated with the following significance:

1. $f(k_i)$ describes the input kinetics from the transdermal device. For a "membrane-controlled" system,[1,2,5,6] $f(k_i)$ consists of both first-order (k^I) and zero-order (k^O) components. The former represents drug release from the contact adhesive, the latter signifies the membrane-limited leaching of drug from the reservoir.[45]

2. k_r reflects the fact that there will be competition for the drug between the patch and the stratum corneum (see above); if the system is well designed, then k_r will be small.

3. k_1 and k_2 are first-order rate constants describing drug transport across the stratum corneum and viable tissue, respectively. k_1 and k_2 are therefore proportional to the corresponding diffusion coefficients through these layers of skin and may be simplistically related to the penetrant molecular weight (M) via Equation 1. (The validity of Equation 1 is assumed for diffusion in the skin.) For benzoic acid, k_1 and k_2 values have been established[40] and hence we may use Equations 3 and 4 to calculate k_1 and k_2 parameters for other penetrants:

$$k_1 = k_1^{BA} (M^{BA}/M)^{1/3} \qquad (3)$$

$$k_2 = k_2^{BA} (M^{BA}/M)^{1/3} \qquad (4)$$

4. The k_3 rate constant describes the affinity of the penetrant for the stratum corneum compared to the viable epidermis. k_3 compensates for the facile estimation of k_1 and allows for greater interaction between penetrant and stratum corneum (thereby producing slower rates of transport out of the horny layer). The ratio k_3/k_2 may be viewed as an effective partition coefficient between stratum corneum and viable epidermis;

the larger the ratio, the longer the penetrant transit time across the outermost skin layer. It has been shown,[46] for most of the compounds analyzed with the kinetic approach, that k_3/k_2 appears to be linearly correlated with the corresponding octanol-water partition coefficient (K) and the relationship

$$k_3/k_2 = K/5 \tag{5}$$

describes this dependence adequately. Thus, if K is known, Equations 3 to 5 can be used to estimate k_1, k_2, and k_3 for any penetrant on the basis of physicochemical properties alone.

5. Finally, k_4 is the elimination rate constant of the drug from the blood. More complicated excretion behavior can be used if necessary. k_4 cannot be predicted but must be measured following i.v. administration of the penetrant.

A series of differential equations characterizes the transdermal absorption of drug from the device into the body according to the scheme shown in Figure 6. As stated, for a membrane-controlled patch, both zero-order and first-order contributions to $f(k_i)$ are expected. Solution of the kinetic expressions in such a situation then leads to the following equation for the concentration of drug in the blood (c);

$$
c = \left\{ \frac{A\ k^0\ k_1 k_2}{V} [1/\alpha\beta\epsilon - \exp(-\alpha t)/(\alpha(\alpha - \beta)(\alpha - \epsilon)) - \exp(-\beta t)/(\beta(\beta - \alpha)(\beta - \epsilon)) \right.
$$

$$
\left. - \exp(-\epsilon t)/(\epsilon(\epsilon - \alpha)(\epsilon - \beta))] \right\} + \left\{ \frac{M_\infty\ k^1 k_1 k_2}{V} [\exp(-\alpha t)/((\beta - \alpha)(\alpha - \omega)(\alpha - \mu)) \right.
$$

$$
- \exp(-\beta t)/((\alpha - \beta)(\beta - \omega)(\beta - \mu)) - \exp(-\omega t)/((\alpha - \omega)(\omega - \beta)(\omega - \mu)) -
$$

$$
\left. \exp(-\mu t)/((\alpha - \mu)(\mu - \beta)(\mu - \omega))] \right\} \tag{6}
$$

The first series of terms in curly brackets is the zero-order contribution, the second is the first-order component. In Equation 6, A is the surface area of the delivery system; M_∞ is the amount of drug in the "priming" contact adhesive; V is the volume of distribution of the drug; and α, β, ϵ, ω and μ are defined by Equations 7 to 9:

$$(\alpha + \beta) = k_2 + k_3 + k_4; \quad \alpha\beta = k_2 k_4 \tag{7}$$

$$\epsilon = k_1 + k_r \tag{8}$$

$$(\omega + \mu) = k^1 + k_r + k_1; \quad \omega\mu = k^1 k_1 \tag{9}$$

To indicate the sensitivity of the rate and extent of transdermal absorption to the physicochemical and pharmacokinetic parameters identified in the model, we have calculated plasma concentration-time profiles as a function of (1) drug molecular weight, (2) effective drug partition coefficient between stratum corneum and viable epidermis, (3) delivery system input rate, and (4) drug biological half-life. The results of the four simulations are shown in Figures 7 to 10; the rate constants used in the calculations are identified in Table 3. To facilitate the presentation we have used only the leading term, i.e., the zero-order contribution in Equation 6, to determine how c varies with time. As will be shown below, the first-order component allows for more rapid attainment of steady-state levels but does not alter the general conclusions discussed here. We observe

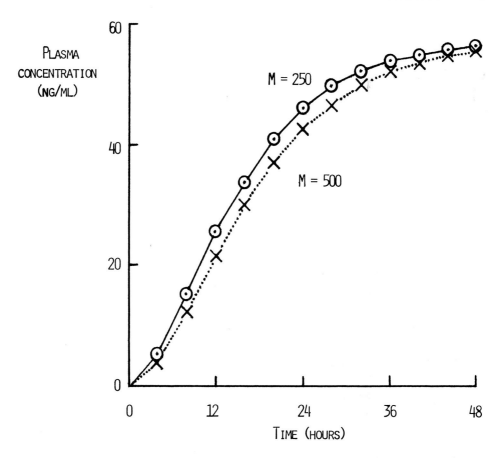

FIGURE 7.   Simulation of plasma concentration-time behavior as a function of penetrant molecular weight (M). The profiles have been calculated using the zero-order term in Equation 6 and the parameters identified in Table 3.

1.   A very weak dependence upon molecular weight; there is almost no difference between the predicted profiles for two drugs having similar properties other than different molecular weights of 250 and 500 (Figure 7). This weak dependence results from the assumption of the validity of Equation 1.

2.   That the plasma level is extremely sensitive to the partitioning characteristics of the drug (Figure 8). The values chosen for k_3 correspond to varying the drug octanol-water partition coefficient from 1 to 1000, i.e., k_3/k_2 varies over the range 0.2 to 200 — see Equation 5. Increasing the lipophilicity of the compound enhances the severity of this function and will considerably prolong the time necessary for steady plasma levels to be reached following transdermal delivery.

3.   Linear dependence of the plateau blood concentration of drug upon the delivery system input rate (k^O) (Figure 9). It should be possible, therefore, to select appropriate delivery kinetics to achieve a desired plasma level. This linearity depends on the relative values of k^O, k_1, and k_2.

4.   Lastly, the biological half-life of the drug (represented in the simulation by k_4) also determines the magnitude of the steady-state plasma concentration and the speed at which this level is reached. Figure 10 shows predicted curves for two molecules differing only in their elimination half-lives (2 hr vs. 12 min).

Thus, pharmacokinetic criteria of major importance may be demonstrated by application

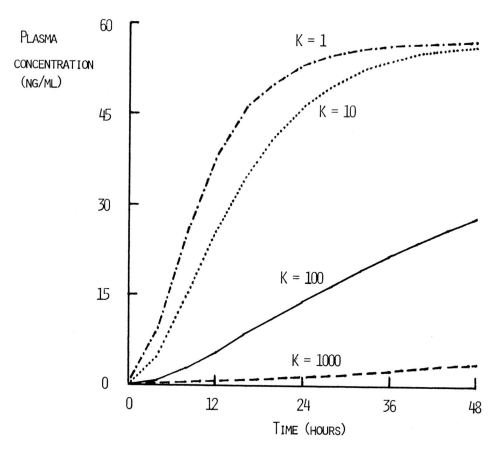

FIGURE 8.   Simulation of plasma concentration-time behavior as a function of penetrant octanol-water partition coefficient (K). The profiles have been calculated using the zero-order term in Equation 6 and the parameters identified in Table 3.

of the simple simulation proposed. In the final section of this chapter, we shall indicate how the kinetic model can bring together the factors discussed here and in the earlier part of the paper. In this way, interpretation and prediction of transdermal drug delivery kinetics are possible and feasible.

V. CONCLUSIONS AND EXAMPLES

A. Nitroglycerin (NTG) and Clonidine

To predict the plasma concentration vs. time profile for NTG and clonidine, we employ Equation 6 with the appropriate values for the parameters required. These parameters are identified in Table 4 and their origin is as follows: k_r is assumed small and of the same value for both drugs; k_1 and k_2 are found from Equations 3 and 4, respectively; k_3 is determined from the octanol-water partition coefficient[47] of the drug using the k_2 value and Equation 5; V and k_4 are obtained from the literature[48] as are the zero-order input kinetics (k^O), the patch area (A), and the "priming" drug dose in the adhesive layer (M_∞).[2,10] Finally, although k^1 (the first-order release kinetics of the drug from the adhesive layer) has not been reported for either NTG or clonidine, we assume that it will have a comparable value to that exhibited by the similarly designed scopolamine therapeutic system.[45] Figures 11 and 12 show the profiles predicted by the derived parameters for NTG and clonidine respectively; the contributions of the zero-order and first-order terms in Equation 6 are indicated. The

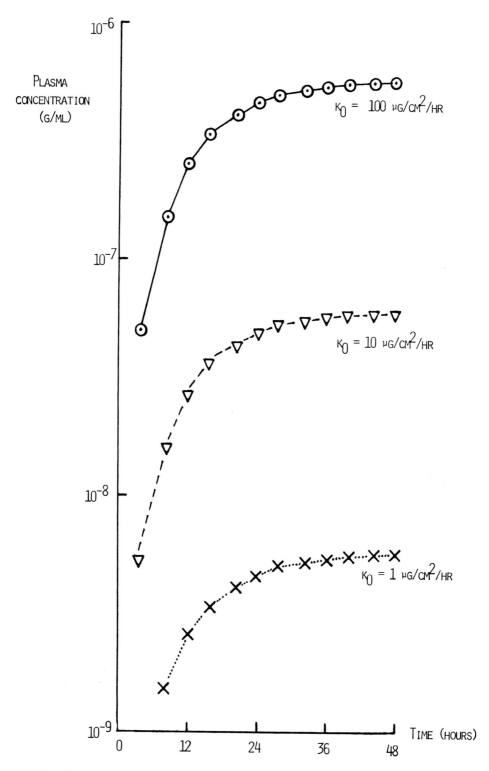

FIGURE 9. Simulation of plasma concentration-time behavior as a function of delivery system input kinetics (k^0). The profiles have been calculated using the zero-order term in Equation 6 and the parameters identified in Table 3. Note that the values of k_1 and k_2 are such that k^0 controls the kinetics.

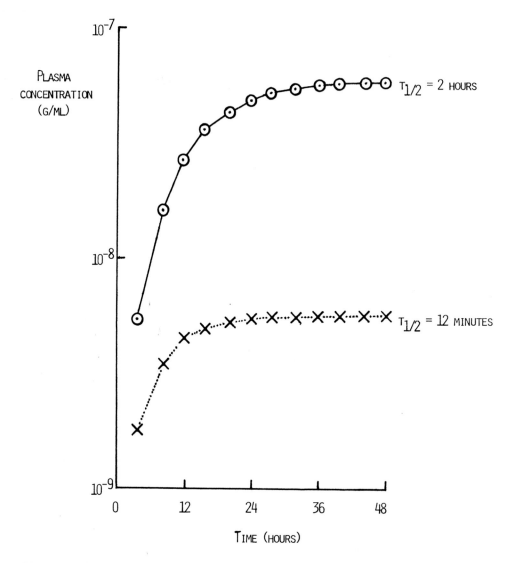

FIGURE 10.   Simulation of plasma concentration-time behavior as a function of drug elimination rate (k_4). The profiles have been calculated using the zero-order term in Equation 6 and the parameters identified in Table 3.

results may be compared with the experimental, in vivo data[9,10] in Figure 2 — the agreement is very reasonable.

We may conclude that the model predicts successfully the plasma concentration of NTG and clonidine following transdermal delivery. While the approach requires known device release characteristics and predetermined drug elimination kinetics and volume of distribution, all transcutaneous kinetic processes are computed directly from physicochemical principles alone. In the remainder of this chapter, we illustrate the utility of the theoretical pathway for screening potential transdermal candidates and for calculating optimum input kinetics in situations for which the administration route seems possible.

B. Indomethacin

Indomethacin is a nonsteroidal anti-inflammatory drug frequently prescribed for chronic treatment situations and requiring (usually) four oral doses per day. *A priori*, therefore, indomethacin would appear to be an attractive transdermal candidate; however, the MEC

Table 3
RATE CONSTANTS EMPLOYED TO CALCULATE THE
SIMULATED PLASMA CONCENTRATION-TIME
PROFILES IN FIGURES 7 TO 10[a]

Figure	k^0 (μg/cm^2/hr)	k_r (hr^{-1})	k_1 (hr^{-1})	k_2 (hr^{-1})	k_3 (hr^{-1})	k_4 (hr^{-1})
7[b]	10	10^{-4}	0.145	2.28	4.56	0.35
	10	10^{-4}	0.115	1.81	3.92	0.35
8	10	10^{-4}	0.145	2.28	0.46	0.35
	10	10^{-4}	0.145	2.28	4.56	0.35
	10	10^{-4}	0.145	2.28	45.6	0.35
	10	10^{-4}	0.145	2.28	456	0.35
9	1	10^{-4}	0.145	2.28	4.56	0.35
	10	10^{-4}	0.145	2.28	4.56	0.35
	100	10^{-4}	0.145	2.28	4.56	0.35
10[c]	10	10^{-4}	0.145	2.28	4.56	0.35
	10	10^{-4}	0.145	2.28	4.56	3.5

[a] The calculations assume A = 10 cm^2 and V = 5ℓ.
[b] For k_1 = 0.145/hr and k_2 = 2.28/hr, M = 250; for k_1 = 0.115/hr and k_2 = 1.81/hr, M = 500.
[c] k_4 = 0.35/hr corresponds to $t_{1/2}$ = 2 hr; k_4 = 3.5/hr corresponds to $t_{1/2}$ = 12 min.

Table 4
PHARMACOKINETIC
PARAMETERS FOR
NITROGLYCERIN AND
CLONIDINE USED TO
CALCULATE THE PREDICTED
PROFILES IN FIGURES 11 AND
12, RESPECTIVELY

	Nitroglycerin	Clonidine
k^0 (μg/cm^2/hr)	36	1.6
k^1 (hr^{-1})	1.3	1.3
k_r (hr^{-1})	10^{-4}	10^{-4}
k_1 (hr^{-1})	0.15	0.15
k_2 (hr^{-1})	2.4	2.4
k_3 (hr^{-1})	53	3.2
k_4 (hr^{-1})	18	0.08
M_∞ (mg)	2	0.5
A (cm^2)	10	5
V (ℓ)	231	147

of this drug is 0.5 to 3 μg/mℓ[48] in plasma, a level which may be suspected to be unattainable via transdermal administration. Simple calculations and application of the kinetic model described above allow the feasibility of the proposal to be tested.

Firstly, if we set the target steady-state plasma concentration (Css) at 1 μg/mℓ, then the necessary input rate (IR) required may be calculated from Equation 10

$$IR = Css \cdot Ke \cdot V \qquad (10)$$

where Ke is the elimination rate constant of the drug (0.28/hr[48]) and V is the volume of distribution (18.2ℓ for a 70 kg adult[48]); hence, IR $\simeq$ 5 mg/hr. Assuming that a 100 cm^2

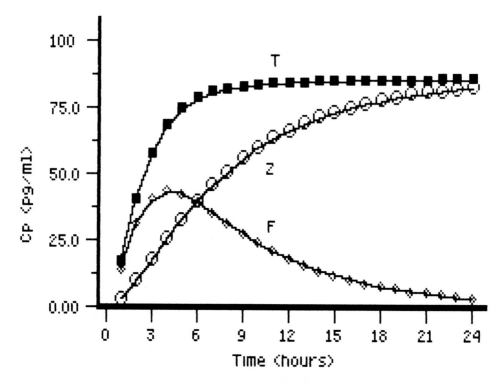

FIGURE 11.   Nitroglycerin: model prediction using Equation 6 and the parameters given in Table 4. Zero-order (Z) and first-order (F) contributions to the total predicted curve (T) are indicated.

patch is reasonable, then the device would have to deliver drug at 50 $\mu g/cm^2/hr$ to be efficacious. These criteria can be tested with the kinetic model. Clearly, drug transport across the skin is likely to be the limiting factor.

We establish parameter values in an equivalent manner to that used in the NTG and clonidine calculations; Table 5 lists these values and indicates their origin. Ignoring, for this illustration, a first-order contribution to the plasma concentration (c) vs. time profile, we can use the leading (zero-order) term in Equation 6 to evaluate c with the parameters in Table 5. The result is shown as curve I in Figure 13. It can be seen that an inordinately long time is necessary for steady-state to be reached and that, even after 120 hr, c is barely one-tenth the target value. This slow ascent to steady state is due to the lipophilic nature of indomethacin and the consequently high stratum corneum/viable tissue partition coefficient. One must recall that k^o and A are such that drug is input at 5 mg/hr; the transdermal patch will contain, therefore, a large quantity of indomethacin.

Can the situation be improved in any way? One possibility is that a penetration enhancer could be used to modify the skin barrier and allow more ready access of drug to the body. In terms of the model, the most facile manner in which the action of an enhancer may be simulated is to increase the value of k_1. Curve II in Figure 13 illustrates the outcome of raising k_1 for indomethacin by a factor of ten (all other parameters maintained at the values shown in Table 5). Only a very slight improvement over curve I is observed. The reason for this insensitivity is the lipophilicity of the drug; the stratum corneum $\rightarrow$ viable epidermis transfer process has thus assumed the major rate-controlling role in the sequence of trans-cutaneous absorption events. The enhancer will be successful, in this case, only if one can alter the relative stratum corneum/viable tissue affinity of the drug. This is shown in curve III of Figure 13 in which we have reduced the ratio k_3/k_2 by an order of magnitude (and maintained k_1 at 1.3/hr); it is now possible for c to approach the target level and to do so more rapidly.

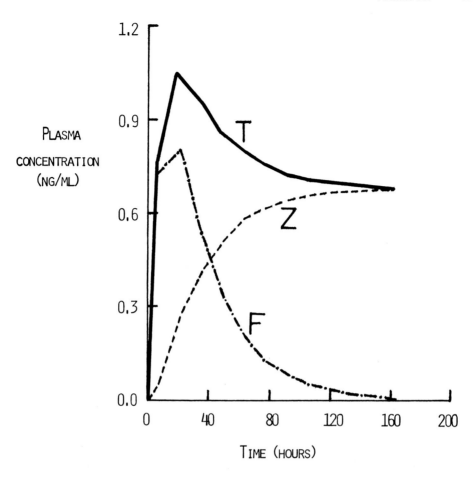

FIGURE 12. Clonidine: model prediction using Equation 6 and the parameters given in Table 4. Zero-order (Z) and first-order (F) contributions to the total predicted curve (T) are indicated.

Table 5
INITIAL PHARMACOKINETIC PARAMETER VALUES FOR INDOMETHACIN REQUIRED TO TEST THE FEASIBILITY OF TRANSDERMAL DELIVERY

Parameter	Value	Comments
k_0 (μg/cm^2/hr)	50	See text
k_r (hr^{-1})	10^{-4}	Consistent with NTG and clonidine
k_1 (hr^{-1})	0.13	From Equation 3 using M = 358
k_2 (hr^{-1})	2.03	From Equation 4 using M = 358
k_3 (hr^{-1})	406	From Equation 5 using k_2 = 2.03 hr^{-1} and K = 1000.[47]
k_4 (hr^{-1})	0.28	Ref. 48
A (cm^2)	100	See text
V (ℓ)	18.2	Ref. 48

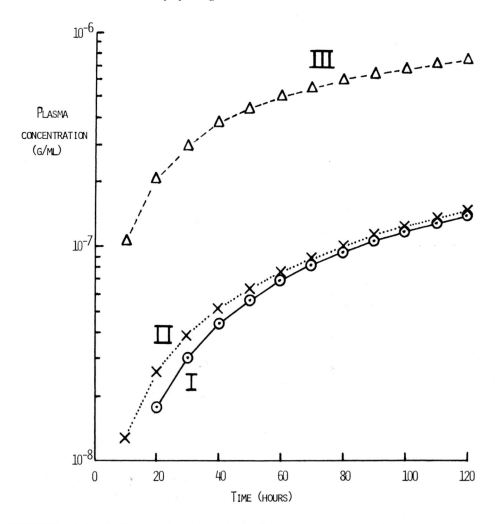

FIGURE 13.   Indomethacin: simulation of plasma concentration (c) vs. time profiles following zero-order trans-
dermal delivery. Curve I is calculated using the leading (zero-order) term in Equation 6 and the parameters in
Table 5. Curve II assumes that a penetration enhancer causes k_1 to be increased by an order of magnitude. Curve
III assumes that the enhancer not only increases k_1 but also reduces the ratio k_3/k_2 by a factor of ten.

Although one would not, at this time, exclude the possibility of transdermal indomethacin
delivery on the basis of the above calculations, it is clear that the objective is difficult. We
have not, for example, explored the effect of a well-conceived loading dose nor have we
investigated the possible utility of a very fast-releasing, shorter-duration, device. Our aim
in this final section has been to illustrate, with practical situations, the way in which the
various drug parameters, identified as important to transdermal delivery, come together to
determine the ultimate feasibility of administration via the skin. While these criteria are
stringent, they are, to a reasonable extent, understood and calculable. We have indicated
one approach (which is by no means a unique possibility) that can apply this comprehension
to achieve both interpretation and prediction of drug input kinetics by the transdermal route.

ACKNOWLEDGMENTS

We thank N. I. H. (GM-33395). Richard H. Guy is the recipient of a Special Emphasis
Research Career Award (1-KO1-0H00017) From N. I. O. S. H.

REFERENCES

1. **Chandrasekaran, S. K. and Shaw, J. E.,** Controlled transdermal delivery, in *Controlled Release of Bioactive Materials,* Baker, R., Ed., Academic Press, New York, 1980, 91.
2. **Good, W. R.,** Transderm-Nitro® controlled delivery of nitroglycerin via the transdermal route, *Drug Dev. Ind. Pharm.,* 9, 647, 1983.
3. **Karim, A.,** Transdermal absorption — a unique opportunity for constant delivery of nitroglycerin, *Drug Dev. Ind. Pharm.,* 9, 671, 1983.
4. **Keith, A. D.,** Polymer matrix considerations for transdermal devices, *Drug Dev. Ind. Pharm.,* 9, 605, 1983.
5. **Weber, M. A., Drayer, J. I. M., Brewer D. D., and Lipson, J. L.,** Transdermal continuous antihypertensive therapy, *Lancet,* 1, 9, 1984.
6. **Laufer, L. R., DeFazio, J. L., Lu, J. K. H., Meldrum, D. R., Eggena, P., Sambhi, M. P., Hershman, J. M., and Judd, H. L.,** *Am. J. Obstet. Gynecol.,* Estrogen replacement therapy by transdermal estradiol administration, 146, 533, 1983.
7. **Needleman, P., Blehm, P. J., Harkey, A. B., Johnson, E. M., and Lang, S.,** The metabolic pathway in the degradation of glyceryl trinitrate, *J. Pharmacol. Exp. Ther.,* 179, 347, 1971.
8. **Noonan, P. K., and Benet, L. Z.,** Formation of mono- and dinitrate metabolites of nitroglycerin following incubation with human blood, *Int. J. Pharm.,* 12, 331, 1982.
9. **Müller, P., Imhof, P. R., Burkart, F., Chu, L.-C., and Gérardin, A.,** Human pharmacological studies of a new transdermal system containing nitroglycerin, *Eur. J. Clin. Pharmacol.,* 22, 473, 1982.
10. **Arndts, D. and Arndts, K.,** Pharmacokinetics and pharmacodynamics of transdermally administered clonidine, *Eur. J. Clin. Pharmacol.,* 26, 79, 1984.
11. **Gilman, A. G., Goodman, L. S., and Gilman, A.,** *The Pharmacological Basis of Therapeutics,* Macmillan, New York, 1980.
12. **Noonan, P. K. and Wester, R. C.,** Cutaneous biotransformations and some pharmacological and toxicological implications, in *Dermatotoxicology,* 2nd ed., Marzulli, F. N. and Maibach, H. I., Eds., Hemisphere, Washington, D.C., 1982, 71.
13. **Wester, R. C., Noonan, P. K., Smeach, S., and Kosobud, L.,** Pharmacokinetics and bioavailability of intravenous and topical nitroglycerin in the rhesus monkey: estimate of percutaneous first-pass metabolism, *J. Pharm. Sci.,* 72, 745, 1983.
14. **Yu, C. D., Fox, J. L., Ho, N. F. H., and Higuchi, W. I.,** Physical model evaluation of topical prodrug delivery — simultaneous transport and bioconversion of vidaribine-5'-valerate. II. Parameter determinations, *J. Pharm. Sci.,* 68, 1347, 1979.
15. **Møllgaard, B., Hoelgaard, A., and Bundgaard, M.,** Pro-drugs as drug delivery systems. XXIII. Improved dermal delivery of 5-fluorouracil through human skin via *N*-acyloxymethyl pro-drug derivatives, *Int. J. Pharm.,* 12, 153, 1982.
16. **Holland, J. M., Kao, J. Y., and Whitaker, M. J.,** A multisample apparatus for kinetic evaluation of skin penetration *in vitro.* The influence of viability and metabolic status of the skin, *Toxicol. Appl. Pharmacol.,* 72, 272, 1984.
17. **Fox, J. L., Yu, C. D., Higuchi, W. I., and Ho, N. F. H.,** General physical model for simultaneous diffusion and metabolism in biological membranes. The computational approach for the steady-state case, *Int. J. Pharm.,* 2, 41, 1979.
18. **Yu, C. D., Fox, J. L., Ho, N. F. H., and Higuchi, W. I.,** Physical model evaluation of topical prodrug delivery — simultaneous transport and bioconversion of vidaribine-5'-valerate. I. Physical model development, *J. Pharm. Sci.,* 68, 1341, 1979.
19. **Hadgraft, J.,** Theoretical aspects of metabolism in the epidermis, *Int. J. Pharm.,* 4, 229, 1979.
20. **Guy, R. H. and Hadgraft, J.,** Percutaneous metabolism with saturable enzyme kinetics, *Int. J. Pharm.,* 11, 187, 1982.
21. **Schaefer, H., Zesch, A., and Stüttgen, G.,** Skin permeability, in *Normal and Pathologic Physiology of the Skin III,* Stüttgen G., Spier, H., and Schwarz, E., Eds., Springer-Verlag, Berlin, 1981, 541.
22. **Scheuplein, R. J. and Blank, I. H.,** Permeability of the skin, *Physiol. Rev.,* 51, 702, 1971.
23. **Scheuplein, R. J., Blank, I. H., Brauner, G. J., and MacFarlane, D. J.,** Percutaneous absorption of steroids, *J. Invest. Dermatol.,* 52, 63, 1969.
24. **Bartek, M. J., LaBudde, J. A., and Maibach, H. I.,** Skin permeability *in vivo:* comparison in rat, rabbit, pig, and man, *J. Invest. Dermatol.,* 58, 114, 1972.
25. **Roberts, M. S., Anderson, R. A., and Swarbrick, J.,** Permeability of human epidermis to phenolic compounds, *J. Pharm. Pharmacol.,* 29, 677, 1977.
26. **Anjo, D. M., Feldmann, R. J., and Maibach, H. I.,** Methods of predicting percutaneous penetration in man, in *Percutaneous Penetration of Steroids.,* Mauvais-Jarvais, P., Wepierre, J., and Vickers, C. F. H., Eds., Academic Press, New York, 1980, 31.

27. **Lien, E. J. and Tong, G. L.,** Physicochemical properties and percutaneous absorption of drugs. *J. Soc. Cosmet. Chem.,* 24, 371, 1973.

28. **Blank, I. H., Scheuplein, R. J., and MacFarlane, D. J.,** Mechanism of percutaneous absorption. III. The effect of temperature on the transport of non-electrolytes across the skin, *J. Invest. Dermatol.,* 49, 582, 1967.

29. **Flynn, G. L., Dürrheim, H., and Higuchi, W. I.,** Permeation of hairless mouse skin. II. Membrane sectioning techniques and influence on alkanol permeabilities, *J. Pharm. Sci.,* 70, 52, 1981.

30. **Michaels, A. S., Chandrasekaran, S. K., and Shaw, J. E.,** Drug permeation through human skin: theory and *in vitro* experimental measurement, *A. I. Ch. E. J.,* 21, 985, 1975.

31. **Barker, N., Hadgraft, J., and Wotton, P. K.,** Facilitated transport across liquid/liquid interfaces and its relevance to drug diffusion across biological membranes. *Farad. Discuss. Chem. Soc.,* 77, 97, 1984.

32. **Inagi, T., Muramatsu, T., Nagai, H., and Terada, H.,** Influence of vehicle composition on the penetration of indomethacin through guinea-pig skin, *Chem. Pharm. Bull.,* 29, 1708, 1981.

33. **Albery, W. J. and Hadgraft, J.,** Percutaneous absorption: theoretical description, *J. Pharm. Pharmacol.,* 31, 129, 1979.

34. **Hadgraft, J.,** The epidermal reservoir; a theoretical approach, *Int. J. Pharm.,* 2, 265, 1979.

35. **Guy, R. H. and Hadgraft, J.,** A theoretical description relating skin penetration to the thickness of the applied medicament. *Int. J. Pharm.,* 6, 321, 1980.

36. **Guy, R. H. and Hadgraft, J.,** Physicochemical interpretation of the pharmacokinetics of percutaneous absorption, *J. Pharmacokinet. Biopharm.,* 11, 189, 1983.

37. **Riegelman, S.,** Pharmacokinetic factors affecting epidermal penetration and percutaneous absorption, *Clin. Pharmacol. Ther.,* 16, 873, 1974.

38. **Wallace, S. M. and Barnett, G.,** Pharmacokinetic analysis of percutaneous absorption: evidence of parallel penetration pathways for methotrexate, *J. Pharmacokinet. Biopharm.,* 6, 315, 1978.

39. **Naito, S.-I. and Tsai, Y.-H.,** Percutaneous absorption of indomethacin from ointment bases in rabbits, *Int. J. Pharm.,* 8, 263, 1981.

40. **Guy, R. H., Hadgraft, J., and Maibach, H. I.,** A pharmacokinetic model for percutaneous absorption. *Int. J. Pharm.,* 11, 119, 1982.

41. **Guy. R. H. and Hadgraft, J.,** Prediction of drug disposition kinetics in skin and plasma following topical application, *J. Pharm. Sci.,* 73, 883, 1984.

42. **Guy, R. H. and Hadgraft, J.,** The prediction of plasma levels of drugs following transdermal application, *J. Controlled Rel.,* 1, 177, 1985.

43. **Guy, R. H. and Hadgraft, J.,** Kinetic analysis of transdermal nitroglycerin delivery, *Pharm. Res.,* 2, 206, 1985.

44. **Guy, R. H. and Hadgraft, J.,** Pharmacokinetic interpretation of the plasma levels of clonidine following transdermal delivery, *J. Pharm. Sci.,* 74, 1016, 1985.

45. **Chandrasekeran, S. K., Bayne, W., and Shaw, J. E.,** Pharmacokinetics of drug permeation through human skin, *J. Pharm. Sci.,* 67, 1370, 1978.

46. **Guy, R. H., Hadgraft, J., and Maibach, H. I.,** Transdermal absorption kinetics: a physicochemical approach, in *Risk Determination for Agricultural Workers from Dermal Exposure to Pesticides,* ACS Symposium Series American Chemical Society, Washington, D.C., in press, 1985.

47. **Hansch, C. and Leo, A. J.,** *Substituent Constants for Correlation Analysis in Chemistry and Biology,* Wiley-Interscience, New York, 1979.

48. **Benet, L. Z. and Sheiner, L. B.,** Design and optimization of dosage regimens; pharmacokinetic data, in *The Pharmacological Basis of Therapeutics,* Gilman, A. G., Goodman, L. S., and Gilman A., Eds., Macmillan, New York, 1980, 1675.

Chapter 2

THERMODYNAMICS OF TRANSDERMAL DRUG DELIVERY

S. Kumar Chandrasekaran

TABLE OF CONTENTS

I. INTRODUCTION

Human skin is very similar to other biological membranes and is a highly organized structure consisting of lipids, protein, and water. Human skin is not homogeneous but it is a mosaic of different functional units differing slightly in structure — highly selective and specialized. However, unlike other biological membranes, human skin is one of the most extensive and readily accessible organs of the human body. Yet, despite the fact that only a fraction of a millimeter of tissue separates the skin surface from the underlying capillary network, we are very well protected against damage by micro- and macromolecular substances as well as the uncontrolled loss of vital biological substances.

An understanding of the nature and origin of the barrier properties of the skin and of the physicochemical characteristics of substances which determine their ability to permeate skin and enter the circulation, would have considerable value to physicians and pharmacologists interested in the use of skin as a route of entry of drugs for the treatment of systemic or dermatologic disorders.

II. PERMEABILITY MECHANISMS

The transport behavior of biological membranes differs in many respects from the more familiar processes in synthetic macroscopic membranes. The differences in diffusional behavior arise from the extremely small membrane thickness involved and this is true irrespective of the specific model used for describing membrane structure. Another major difference is the more complex nature of the transport processes, in particular, their heavy reliance on facilitated diffusion. Finally, there is the phenomenon of active transport, for which there is as yet no counterpart in nonliving systems. Active transport is a special case of carrier or facilitated transport in which solutes are moved against electrochemical gradients directly by means of energy releasing chemical reactions.

In the case of skin, the work of Scheuplein and co-workers ultimately clarified the focus and origin of the molecular permeability characteristics and established it to be a passive rather than a biologically active property.[1-4] Through their studies of the permeability of excised human skin in vitro to a large number of substances, they were able to show conclusively that the principal barrier to permeation is provided by the stratum corneum.

By separating epidermis from the underlying dermis enzymatically removing the unkeratinized live epidermal layer, and then subsequently measuring the permeabilities of the stratum corneum and dermis independently, it was shown that the stratum corneum is at least three, and frequently as much as five orders of magnitude less permeable to most substances than the dermis. Moreover, the permeability of the entire epidermis was found to be indistinguishable from that of the stratum corneum alone. Scheuplein and his collaborators thereby modeled the skin as a three layer laminate of stratum corneum, epidermis, and dermis with permeation occurring by Fickian diffusion of the penetrating species through the three layers in series array.[1-4] Since the dominant resistance to permeation of most compounds is offered by the stratum corneum, the gradient in penetrant concentration across the entire skin is, for all practical purposes, localized within the stratum corneum.

III. THERMODYNAMICS OF DRUG PERMEATION

In a typical in vitro skin permeation experiment, a sample of skin of essentially uniform thickness is contacted on its external (stratum corneum) surface with a solution of penetrant of known concentration on its internal (dermis) surface with water, physiological saline, or Ringers solution, and the steady-state rate of transport of penetrant across the tissue is measured by appropriate means.

In this manner, the transdermal flux of penetrant J, in, for example, $\mu g/cm^2/hr$, can be computed with little ambiguity. If one assumes the tissue layer to be homogeneous and that the penetrant permeates by simple molecular diffusion, then the flux J can be represented by Fick's equation:

$$J = -D_M \frac{dC_M}{dx} \simeq D_M \frac{\Delta C_M}{t} \qquad (1)$$

where D_M is the penetrant diffusivity in the membrane, ΔC_M is the penetrant concentration decrement across the membrane, and t is the membrane thickness. In most cases, the penetrant concentration at the downstream boundary is maintained at or close to zero, whereupon

$$J \simeq D_M \frac{C_{M(1)}}{t} \qquad (2)$$

where $C_{M(1)}$ is the concentration of penetrant in the tissue contacting the source of the penetrant. Since the direct determination of $C_{M(1)}$ is usually difficult, it is common practice to express Equation 2 in the form

$$J = \overline{P} \left(\frac{C_1}{t} \right) \qquad (3)$$

where $\overline{P}$ is the specific permeability of the membrane to the penetrant, and C_1 is the penetrant concentration in the solution contacting the membrane. Simultaneous solution of Equations 2 and 3 yields

$$\overline{P} = D_M \frac{C_{M(1)}}{C_1} = k_M D_M \qquad (4)$$

where k_M is the partition coefficient of the penetrant between membrane and contacting solution.

If both k_M and D_M are independent of penetrant concentration, then it is obvious from Equation 3 that the transmembrane flux will be directly proportional to the penetrant concentration in the contacting solution.

The use of $\overline{P}$ as defined in Equation 4 to characterize the permeability of skin (or any membrane) to a specific penetrant, while of customary practice among researchers in skin permeation, is confusing and ambiguous since its magnitude is determined not only by the properties of the penetrant and its interaction with the tissue, but also by the solvent used in preparing the penetrant solution. This is true even if the solvent has no influence on the transport processes occurring within the membrane. Since most drugs of interest in skin penetration are solids or liquids of finite water solubility and since the permeability of skin when in saturation equilibrium with liquid water is of primary importance, we can define a more useful term for characterizing skin permeability:

$$J_{max} = \overline{P} \frac{C^*}{t} = D_M \frac{C^*_M}{t} \qquad (5)$$

where J_{max} is the maximum flux of penetrant through the skin when contacted with a saturated aqueous penetrant solution of concentration C^*.

Since C^*_M is the penetrant concentration within the membrane when in saturation equilibrium with unit activity penetrant, this value is solvent independent (so long as the solvent does not solvate the membrane), and thus the product $[J_{max}(t)]$ is truly descriptive of the permeability of the membrane to a specific penetrant.

If, furthermore, it can be assumed that, for any penetrant or solvent

$$\alpha = C/C^* \tag{6}$$

and

$$C_M = \alpha\, C^*_M \tag{7}$$

where α is the activity of the penetrant in solution when its concentration is C, then Equation 5 can be rewritten as

$$J = J_{max} \frac{C}{C^*} = \overline{P} \frac{C}{t} = D_M \frac{C^*_M\, C}{C^*\, t} \tag{8}$$

We can now define the term $\overline{J}$ as the normalized flux

$$\overline{J} = \frac{J}{C} = \frac{J_{max}}{C^*} = \frac{\overline{P}}{t} \tag{9}$$

where, it is clear that the permeation flux will be proportional to the penetrant concentration in the contacting solution up to the saturation limit. The term $[J_{max}(t)]$ may be regarded as the intrinsic permeability of the membrane to a given penetrant.

In dealing with steady-state permeation through whole skin, Scheuplein and others have treated the tissue as a trilayer laminate, each layer of which transmits penetrant by normal Fickian diffusion with partition equilibrium of penetrant being maintained at the interlayer boundaries. Under these assumptions, the flux across the tissue is given simply by

$$\frac{Jt_0}{C} = \overline{P}_0 = \frac{t_0}{\dfrac{t_1}{P_1} + \dfrac{t_2}{P_2} + \dfrac{t_3}{P_3}} \tag{10}$$

or

$$J_{max(0)} = \frac{1}{\dfrac{1}{J_{max(1)}} + \dfrac{1}{J_{max(2)}} + \dfrac{1}{J_{max(3)}}} \tag{11}$$

where the subscripts (1), (2), and (3) refer to the individual layers (stratum corneum, epidermis, dermis) of the laminate and (0) to the entire laminate. Since, as pointed out above, the permeation barrier imposed by the stratum corneum is by far the greatest, Equations 10 and 11 reduce to

$$\frac{Jt_0}{C} = \overline{P}_0 = \overline{P}_S \frac{t_0}{t_S} \tag{12}$$

and

$$J_{max(0)} = J_{max(S)} \tag{13}$$

where S refers to the stratum corneum.

Hence, measurement of the permeability of whole skin to specific penetrants yields for all practical purposes the rate of penetration of the stratum corneum alone. It is, therefore, appropriate to attempt to characterize the stratum corneum per se in an effort to explain and predict drug and other penetrant transport through intact skin.

An idealized model of the stratum corneum is suggested by experimental observations that the tissue is capable of soaking up to six times its dry weight in water, with a very great increase in permeability upon lipid extraction. We postulate that the tissue consists of an essentially parallel array of thin plates, each consisting mostly of protein, which are separated from one another by thin layers of interstitial lipoidal material. The interstitial lipid rich phase is the continuous phase of the matrix, whereas the proteinaceous phase is discontinuous and by far the larger volume fraction of the tissue.

For any permeating species, there are only two routes for penetration of the barrier: one requires alternate transit through protein and lipid phases, and the other, transit solely through the continuous lipid phase. The overall permeability of the composite barrier can be quantitatively related to the specific transport properties of the two phases and to their geometric configuration.

Within each phase, the permeating species is assumed to have a characteristic solubility (proportional to its local thermodynamic activity) and diffusivity. The details of the mathematical derivation have been previously described by Michaels et al., and the overall steady-state permeability of the tissue is expressed in Equation 14:

$$\bar{J} = 0.135\sigma \frac{D_L}{D_P} \left[\frac{1.16 + 0.0017(\sigma D_L/D_P)}{0.16 + (\sigma D_L/D_P)} \right] \tag{14}$$

where $\bar{J} = J_{S(max)}/C^*$. Here σ is the lipid/protein partition coefficient, and D_L and D_P are the diffusion constants in the lipid and protein phases, respectively.

Equation 14 can be further simplified as follows:

$$\text{Case I:} \quad \sigma D_L/D_P \text{ very small} \tag{15}$$

$$\bar{J} \simeq 0.98 \frac{\sigma D_L}{D_P} \tag{16}$$

$$\text{Case II:} \quad \sigma D_L/D_P \text{ very large}$$

$$\bar{J} \simeq 2.3 \times 10^{-4} \frac{\sigma D_L}{D_P}$$

The theoretical plot of Equation 14 depicting the variation of the normalized drug flux $\bar{J}$ with $\sigma D_L/D_P$ is shown in Figure 1.

The quantity σ (lipid/protein partition coefficient) can, for most drugs, be approximated by the experimentally determined oil/water partition coefficient, so long as the oil phase used in the measurement is of cohesive energy density not unlike that of the lipid phase of the stratum corneum.

Thus, drugs that are either exceedingly insoluble in water and/or have very low oil solubility will display low rates of skin permeation. Conversely, drugs that are both highly water soluble and have a strong tendency to partition into oils will display relatively high rates of skin permeation.

For ionogenic drug compounds the process of skin permeation is further complicated by the simultaneous presence of both ionized and nonionic species in solution, each of which

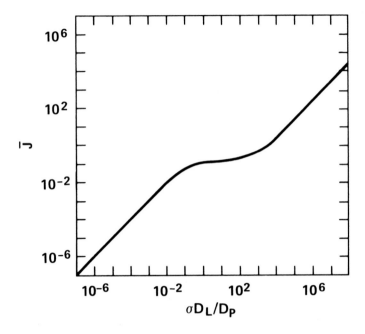

FIGURE 1.   Theoretical variation of normalized transdermal flux with $\sigma D_L/D_P$.

permeates through the skin at different rates. If it is assumed that each species migrates through the skin by simple diffusion at a rate governed solely by its own concentration gradient and unaltered by the presence of other species, we can correlate the total flux of drug in terms of the sum of the fluxes of the species present and their respective concentrations and concentration gradient.

If a drug is a weak base, its behavior in solution can be represented by

$$BH^+ \leftrightarrows B + H^+$$

where BH^+ is the protonated, ionized form of the compound and B is the unionized, free-base form.

The relative concentrations of ionized and unionized forms in solution are, of course, governed by the equilibrium relationship

$$K_A = \frac{(C_B)(C_{H^+})}{(C_{BH^+})} \tag{17}$$

If we define $C_{B(0)}$ as the total concentration of the compound present in solution in all forms, then Equation 17 can be written as

$$\frac{(C_B)}{(C_{BH^+})} = \frac{(C_B)}{(C_{B(0)} - C_B)} = \frac{K_A}{(C_{H^+})} \tag{17a}$$

or

$$\frac{C_B}{C_{B(0)}} = \frac{K_A/(C_{H^+})}{1 + K_A/(C_{H^+})} \tag{17b}$$

Whereupon, the absolute and relative concentrations of the drug in the two forms can be computed by knowing the total drug concentration, the acid ionization constant of the compound K_A, and the pH of the solution.

If we assume that the transdermal flux of each species is determined by

$$\frac{J_B t_S}{C_B} = \overline{P}_B \tag{18}$$

$$\frac{J_{BH^+} t_S}{C_{BH^+}} = \overline{P}_{BH^+} \tag{19}$$

then

$$J_{B(0)} = J_B + J_{BH^+} = \frac{\overline{P}_B C_B + \overline{P}_{BH^+} C_{BH^+}}{t_S} \tag{20}$$

or

$$\frac{J_{B(0)} t_S}{C_{B(0)}} = \overline{P}_B \frac{C_B}{C_{B(0)}} + \overline{P}_{BH^+} \frac{C_{BH^+}}{C_{B(0)}} \tag{21}$$

or

$$\frac{J_{B(0)} t_S}{C_{B(0)}} = \frac{\overline{P}_B + \overline{P}_{BH^+} (C_{H^+} + /K_A)}{(1 + C_{H^+} + /K_A)} \tag{22}$$

From Equation 22, it is evident that if $(K_A/C_{H^+}) \gg 1$,

$$\frac{J_{B(0)} t_S}{C_{B(0)}} \rightarrow \overline{P}_B$$

and if $(K_A/C_{H^+}) \rightarrow 0$,

$$\frac{J_{B(0)} t_S}{C_{B(0)}} \rightarrow \overline{P}_{BH^+}$$

and if $C_{H^+} = K_A$,

$$\frac{J_{B(0)} t_S}{C_{B(0)}} = \frac{\overline{P}_B + \overline{P}_{BH^+}}{2}$$

It is also clear from Equation 22 that at constant solution pH, the transdermal permeation rate should be proportional to the total drug concentration in the contacting solution.

The quantities $\overline{P}_B$ and $\overline{P}_{BH^+}$ in Equation 22 should, from Equation 15, be equivalent to

$$\frac{\overline{P}_B}{t_S} = \sigma B \frac{D_{L(B)}}{D_{P(B)}} \tag{23}$$

and

$$\frac{\overline{P}_{BH^+}}{t_S} = \sigma(BH^+)\frac{D_{L(BH^+)}}{D_{P(BH^+)}} \tag{24}$$

If it is assumed that the diffusion coefficients of the drug in the protein and lipid phases of the stratum corneum are the same for the ionized and unionized forms, then it follows that

$$\frac{\overline{P}_B}{P_{BH^+}} \simeq \frac{\sigma(B)}{\sigma(BH^+)} \tag{25}$$

This indicates that the specific permeabilities of the skin to the ionized and unionized forms of the drug are in the ratio of their oil/water partition coefficients. Since the free energy change associated with the transfer of an ion pair from an aqueous (high dielectric constant) to an oil (low dielectric constant) phase is invariably greater than that for transfer of a neutral molecule, one should expect that $\sigma(B)>>(\sigma BH^+)$ whereupon $\overline{P}_B>>\overline{P}_{BH^+}$. Hence, one should also expect the specific permeability of skin to the unionized form of a drug to be substantially greater than that of the ionized form. However, the maximum rate of permeation is also determined by the maximum achievable concentration of the species in water; hence

$$\frac{J_{max(B)}}{J^{(BH^+)}_{(max)}} = \frac{\overline{P}_B C^* Aq(B)}{P_{BH^+} C^* Aq(BH^+)} \simeq \frac{\sigma(B)}{\sigma(BH^+)}\frac{C^* Aq(B)}{C^* Aq(BH^+)} \tag{26}$$

Thus, if the water solubility of the free base, unionized form of the drug is much less than that of its ionized salt, its rate of permeation in unionized form may be lower than that of its salt, even though the intrinsic permeability of the skin to the free base may be much greater.

For drugs that display low permeability through skin, significant sorption of the drug by the skin may greatly delay the establishment of steady-state permeation conditions.

We have attempted to reconcile the disparity between steady-state and time lag diffusivities using the "dual mode sorption model," which has been extensively utilized to explain the equilibrium sorption data for gases in polymers. The model postulates that sorption occurs by two mechanisms: the first mechanism being a simple dissolution that produces mobile and freely diffusible molecules and the second being an adsorption process producing non-mobile molecules that do not participate in the diffusion process.[6]

The total concentration of drug in the skin is thus assumed to be composed of two parts:

$$C_T = C_D + C_I \tag{27}$$

The mobile drug concentration, C_D, can be adequately expressed in the proportionality:

$$C_D = k_D C \tag{28}$$

On the other hand, the concentration of immobilized drug, C_I, can be represented by an adsportion isotherm of the Langmuir form:

$$C_I = \frac{C_I^* bC}{1 + bC} \tag{29}$$

Assuming that exchange between mobile and immobile drug molecules is rapid compared with the diffusion process, the steady-state diffusion coefficient, D_{SS}, can be related to the apparent time lag diffusion coefficient, D_{TL}:

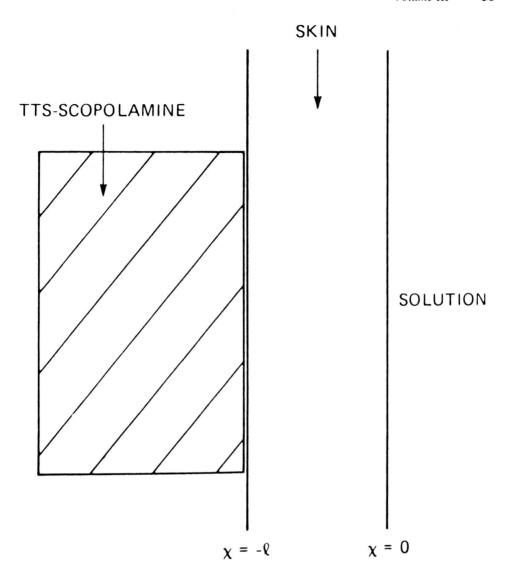

FIGURE 2. Diagram of system placed on skin.

$$\frac{D_{SS}}{D_{TL}} = \frac{\left\{1 + 6\,C_I^*d\left[\dfrac{0.5(bC)^2 + bC - (1 + bC)\,\ell n(1 + bC)}{(bC)^3}\right]\right\}}{\left[1 + \dfrac{C_I^*d}{(1 + bC)^2}\right]} \tag{30}$$

IV. THERMODYNAMICS OF CONTROLLED DELIVERY

The delivery of a drug from a transdermal system into and across human skin in vivo can be modeled, assuming that drug transport occurs by normal Fickian diffusion, with partition equilibrium of penetrant being maintained at the interlayer boundaries.[7]

With reference to Figure 2 and the assumptions that infinite sink conditions are maintained on the dermal side of the skin, the temporal variation of the drug concentration in the skin is given by Equation 31:

$$\frac{\partial C_D}{\partial t} = \frac{D}{\left[1 + \dfrac{C_I^* b/k_D}{(1 + C_D b/k_D)^2}\right]} \frac{\partial^2 C_D}{\partial x^2} \tag{31}$$

with boundary conditions:

$$C_D = 0 \qquad \text{at x and t} = 0$$
$$C_D = 0 \qquad \text{at x} = 0 \text{ and t}$$
$$\frac{dC_D}{dx}\bigg|_{x=-l} = f(t) \qquad \text{at x} = -l \text{ and t} > 0$$

$$\frac{dC_D}{dx}\bigg|_{x=-l} = \frac{-D}{\left[1 + \dfrac{C_I^* b/k_D}{(1 + C_D b/k_D)^2}\right]}$$

where $f(t) = G + He^{-ht}$, the temporal pattern of drug delivery from the device in the absence of skin.

To provide mathematical simplicity to obtain an analytical solution, it is assumed that, based on experimental data:

$$\frac{C_I^* b/k_D}{(1 + C_D b/k_D)^2} \simeq \text{constant} = R \tag{32}$$

Under these conditions, the analytical solution of Equation 31 is

$$C_D = \frac{2}{l} \sum_{n=1}^{\infty} (-1)^{n-1} \exp[-\alpha(2n - 1)^2 t](2n - 1)^2 t$$

$$\sin \frac{(2n - 1)\pi x}{2l} \left[\frac{G}{\alpha(2n - 1)^2} (\exp[(2n - 1)^2 \alpha t] - 1)\right.$$

$$\left. + \frac{H}{(2n - 1)^2 \alpha - h} (\exp[(2n - 1)^2 \alpha - h] t - 1)\right] \tag{33}$$

where $\alpha = \pi^2 D/[4L^2(R + 1)]$.

From mass balance considerations, the drug accumulation in the systemic circulation equals the input of drug in vivo minus the excretion of drug in vivo and is given by:

$$\frac{V dC_P}{dt} = \frac{D}{R + 1} \frac{dC_D}{dx}\bigg|_{x=0} - k_E C_P V \tag{34}$$

where dC_D/dx is the derivative of Equation 33 with respect to x. Therefore:

$$\frac{V dC_P}{dt} = k_E C_P V = \frac{4}{\pi} \alpha \sum_{n=1}^{\infty} (-1)^{n-1} (2n - 1) \exp[-\alpha(2n - 1)^2 t]$$

$$\times \left[\frac{G}{\alpha(2n - 1)^2} (\exp[(2n - 1)^2 \alpha t] - 1) + \frac{H}{(2n - 1)^2 \alpha - h} (\exp[(2n - 1)^2 \alpha - h] t - 1)\right] \tag{35}$$

The solution of Equation 35 is given by:

$$C_pV = \frac{4}{\pi} \alpha e \, k_E t \sum_{n=1}^{\infty} (-1)^{n-1} (2n-1)$$

$$\times \left[\frac{G}{\alpha(2n-1)^2} \left(\frac{e \, k_E t}{k_E} - \frac{\exp[k_E - \alpha(2n-1)^2] \, t}{k_E - \alpha(2n-1)^2} - \frac{1}{k_E} \right. \right.$$

$$\left. + \frac{1}{k_E - \alpha(2n-1)^2} \right) + \frac{H}{(2n-1)^2 \, \alpha - h} \left(\frac{\exp(k_E - h) \, t}{k_E - h} \right.$$

$$\left. \left. - \frac{e^{[k_E - \alpha(2n-1)^2]t}}{k_E - \alpha(2n-1)^2} - \frac{1}{k_E - h} + \frac{1}{k_E - \alpha(2n-1)^2} \right) \right] \qquad (36)$$

Under transdermal drug administration, the model predicts that the urinary drug excretion rate is given by:

$$R_E = \frac{4}{\pi} \alpha k_E \sum_{n=1}^{\infty} (-1)^{n-1} (2n-1)$$

$$\left[\frac{G}{\alpha(2n-1)^2} \left(\frac{1}{k_E} - \frac{e^{-\alpha(2n-1)^2 t}}{k_E - \alpha(2n-1)^2} - \frac{e^{-k_E t}}{k_E} \right. \right.$$

$$\left. + \frac{e^{-k_E t}}{k_E - \alpha(2n-1)^2} \right) + \frac{H}{(2n-1)^2 \, \alpha - h} \left(\frac{e^{-ht}}{k_E - h} \right.$$

$$\left. \left. - \frac{e^{-\alpha(2n-1)^2 t}}{k_E - \alpha(2n-1)^2} - \frac{e^{-k_E t}}{k_E - h} + \frac{e^{-k_E t}}{k_E - \alpha(2n-1)^2} \right) \right] \qquad (37)$$

In the limit of large values for time t:

$$R_E = \frac{4\alpha}{\pi} k_E \sum_{n=1}^{\infty} (-1)^{n-1} \frac{G}{(2n-1) \, \alpha k_E} = G \qquad (38)$$

which implies that, under steady-state conditions, the urinary drug excretion rate will be constant and equal to the steady-state drug input rate. It has been assumed in this model that all elimination occurs by excretion. If this assumption had not been made, the steady-state excretion rate would equal the fraction of drug excreted times the steady-state drug input.

After the termination of transdermal drug administration, assuming a linear drug concentration gradient in the skin, the urinary drug excretion rate is given by Equation 39:

$$R_E{}^* = \alpha \beta k_E \sum_{n=0}^{\infty} \frac{1}{(2n+1)} \sin \left(\frac{2n+1}{2} \right) \times \pi \left[\frac{e^{-(2n+1)^2 \alpha t} - e^{-k_E t}}{k_E - (2n+1)^2 \, \alpha} \right] \qquad (39)$$

where $\beta = (16 \, l \, C_D{}^*)/\pi^3$.

V. EXPERIMENTAL RESULTS

A. Steady-State Permeation

The experimentally measured steady-state permeation rates for a variety of drug compounds are shown in Table 1; also tabulated are drug/water solubilities, mineral oil/water partition coefficient, pK values, where applicable, donor solution pH, and computed values of normalized flux. Permeability measurements for each drug were performed on skin samples

Table 1
SUMMARY OF EXPERIMENTAL RESULTS

Drug	Source of radiolabel drug[a]	Radiolabel	Water solubility at 30°C (mg/mℓ)	Mineral oil/water partition coeff at 30°C	pK	Solution pH	No. of skin donors	Number of permeation experiments	Range of $J_{S(max)}$ at 30°C ($\mu g/cm^2/hr$)	Avg. $J_{S(max)}$ at 30°C ($\mu g/cm^2/hr$)	Avg. J at 30°C (cm/hr × 10³)
Ephedrine	NEN	^{14}C	50	1.0	9.65	10.8	3	8	250—400	300	6.0
Diethylcarbamazine			800	0.064		10.0	2	6	83—120	100	0.13
Nitroglycerin			1.3	10		—	2	4	10—25	13	11
Scopolamine	ICN	^3H	75	0.026	7.35	9.6	5	10	2.0—8.0	3.8	0.05
Chlorpheniramine	ICN	^3H	1.6	0.46	9.1	10.3	4	8	2.9—3.9	3.5	2.2
Fentanyl	McNeal	^3H	0.2	200		8.0	5	10	0.8—3.8	2.0	10
Atropine	A/S	^3H	2.4	0.006		8.0	2	5	0.01—0.05	0.02	0.0086
Estradiol	NEN	^3H	0.003	12		7.0	4	8	0.01—0.03	0.016	5.2
Ouabain	NEN	^3H	10	0.00026		7.0	2	4	0.005—0.02	0.008	0.00078
Digitoxin	NEN	^3H	0.01	0.014		7.0	1	2	0.00012—0.00014	0.00013	0.013

[a]   A/S = Amersham/Searle; NEN = New England Nuclear Corporation; ICN = International Chemical & Nuclear Corp.

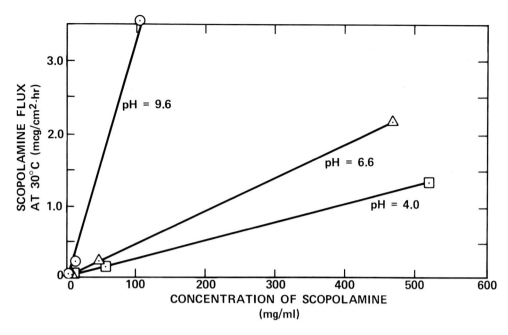

FIGURE 3.   Effect of concentration and pH on scopolamine flux through human skin.

Table 2
PERMEATION BEHAVIOR OF SCOPOLAMINE
FROM SATURATED AQUEOUS SOLUTIONS

Drug form	Skin	Skin thickness (cm)	Steady-state flux ($\mu g/cm^2/hr$)
Free base	Whole skin	0.0953	6.0
	Epidermis	0.0051	6.7
	Dermis	0.0889	1342
Salt	Whole skin	0.0953	0.8
	Dermis	0.0889	5710

from several subjects and the reported range in-flux values thus reflects the variability in skin permeability between individuals. The differences in maximum skin transport rates among drugs are enormous — the highest (~ 300 $\mu g/cm^2/hr$) being ephedrine and the lowest ($\sim 1.3 \times 10^{-4}$ $\mu g/cm^2/hr$) for digitoxin.

B. Scopolamine

Scopolamine, which was first extracted from the belladonna plant, is an alkaloid with a pK of 7.35; water solubility of the base is 75 mg/mℓ at 30°C and of the hydrobromide salt, 520 mg/mℓ. The transdermal flux of scopolamine as a function of concentration and pH of the aqueous drug solution contacting the stratum corneum surface of the tissue is shown in Figure 3. The in vitro flux of scopolamine at constant pH shows a linear increase with increasing concentration. Under saturation conditions, at pH 9.6 where the drug is present almost entirely as the free base, the maximum flux is attained, indicating that the base form is by far more skin permeable than the ionized salt form.

The permeation rate of scopolamine from saturated aqueous donor solutions through epidermis, dermis, and whole skin is presented in Table 2. For the scopolamine base, permeation through whole skin occurs at a rate similar to that through epidermis alone, confirming that the epidermis or stratum corneum offers the principal resistance to the

Table 3
PERMEATION AND IMMOBILIZATION OF SCOPOLAMINE IN EPIDERMIS

Skin	Scopolamine in donor (mg/mℓ)	Epidermal thickness (cm)	Scopolamine in epidermis (mg/mℓ)	Scopolamine steady-state flux (μg/cm²/hr)
Thigh	4.6	0.0106	16.9	4.7
	16.9		25.7	15.5
Postauricular	4.6	0.0084	7.4	10.0
	16.9		13.9	24.3

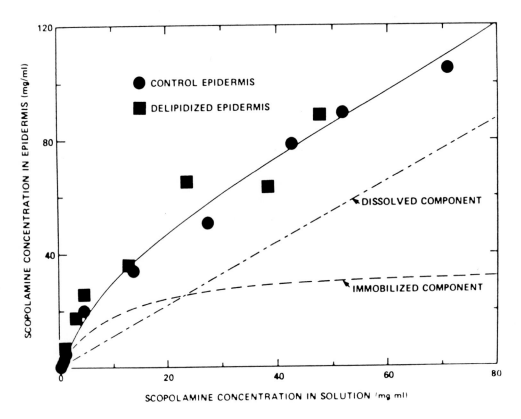

FIGURE 4.   Scopolamine sorption isotherm in human epidermis in vitro.

transdermal permeation of scopolamine. The permeation rate through dermis is several orders of magnitude greater than that through intact skin; in fact, the salt form of the drug is more permeable, possibly due to its increased water solubility compared to the free base.

Further experiments showed that the permeation rate of scopolamine base through intact epidermis varied depending upon the skin site from which the tissue was excised. In Table 3, the steady-state flux of scopolamine is shown as a function of drug concentration in contact with the stratum corneum surface of skin excised both from the thigh and postauricular region of the same cadaver. It is apparent that the postauricular region is the more permeable to transport of scopolamine.

An equilibrium sorption isotherm for scopolamine base in both the control and lipid extracted epidermis is shown in Figure 4. Prior to the sorption experiment, the tissue was extracted for 3 hr with a chloroform/methanol mixture and subsequently rehydrated without

Table 4
EFFECT OF DELIPIDIZATION ON
SCOPOLAMINE DIFFUSION
COEFFICIENTS

Tissue	Average steady-state diffusion coefficient (cm²/sec)
Control epidermis	4×10^{-10}
Delipidized epidermis	2×10^{-7}

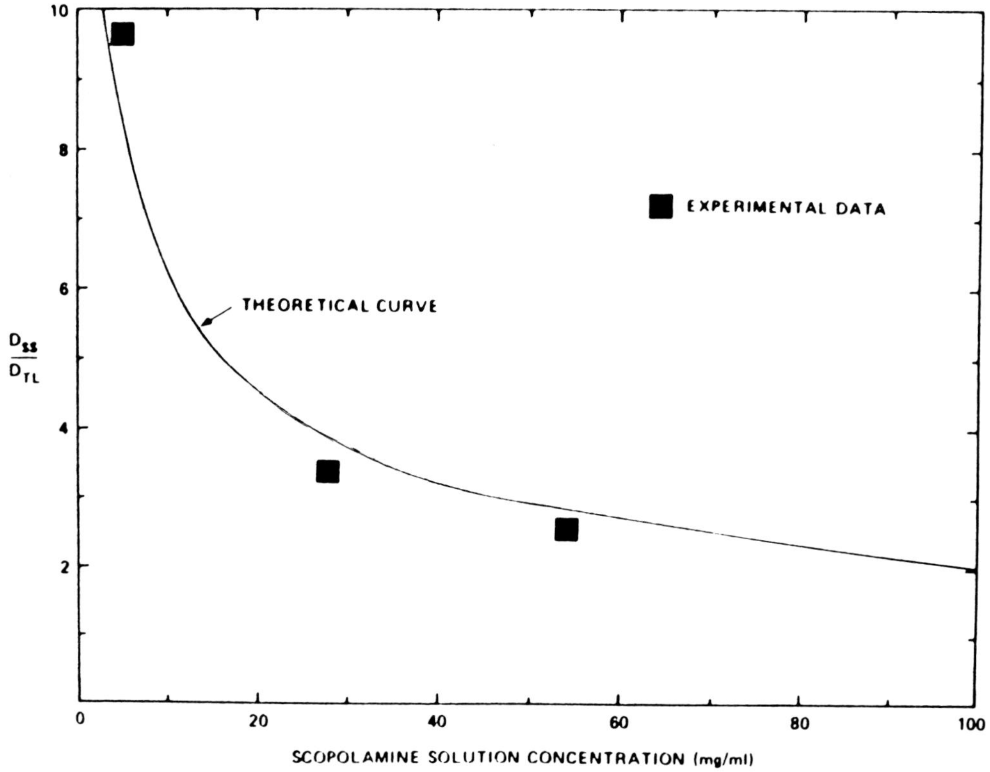

FIGURE 5.   Variation of D_{SS}/D_{TL} with scopolamine concentration.

detectable morphological or mechanical alterations. Selective removal of the lipid components apparently has no effect on the equilibrium sorption behavior of the tissue. Using the dual mode sorption model, the isotherm can be split into the dissolved and immobilized components and the values of the constants K_D, C^*_I, and b are, respectively, 1.1, 36.0 mg/mℓ, and 0.11 mℓ/mg. Steady-state diffusivities were determined by dividing the measured steady-state flux by the computed gradient of dissolved drug (Table 4). Lipid extraction of the epidermis prior to permeation measurements results in a 500-fold increase in steady-state diffusivity.

A comparison is made between the ratio of the steady state to time lag diffusivities measured experimentally as a function of concentration, and the ratio predicted by using Equation 30; the agreement between theory and experiment is good (Figure 5).

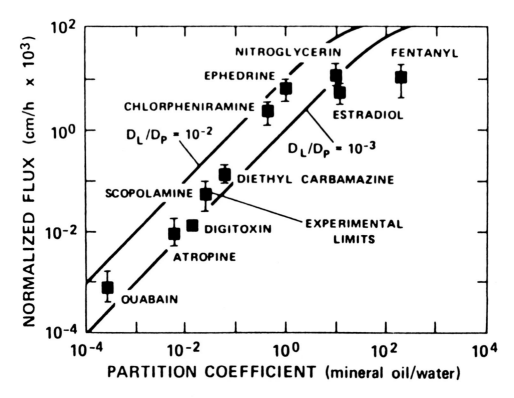

FIGURE 6.   Variation of normalized transdermal flux with partition coefficient.

Table 5
NORMALIZED DRUG FLUXES THROUGH
HUMAN SKIN IN VITRO

	Normalized flux (cm/hr $\times$ 10⁴)	
Drug	Base form ($\overline{P}_B/t_S$)	Ionized form ($\overline{P}_{BH+}/t_S$)
Ephedrine	60	3.3
Scopolamine	0.5	0.03
Chlorpheniramine	22	0.08

C. Permeability Correlation

The normalized transdermal fluxes for a variety of drug compounds — for amino drugs, the values are those of the free bases — are plotted against the respective mineral oil/water partition coefficients (Figure 6). The vertical bars represent the scatter of the permeability values between individual skin samples. Also plotted in Figure 6 are two numerical solutions to Equation 14, on the assumption that the lipid/protein partition coefficient is equal to the measured mineral oil/water partition coefficient and for values of D_L/D_P of 10^{-2} and 10^{-3}. The region between the two lines envelopes most of the experimental data and the best theoretical fit is obtained for a value of D_L/D_P of 2×10^{-3}. We can now conclude that the lipid/protein partition coefficient can be approximated by the mineral oil/water partition coefficient and that the diffusivity of the drug base in the lipid phase is about 500 times lower than its diffusion coefficient in the protein phase.

If the normalized flux values for the ionized forms of ephedrine, scopolamine, and chlorpheniramine (Table 5) are made to fit the correlation of Figure 5 for the free base forms,

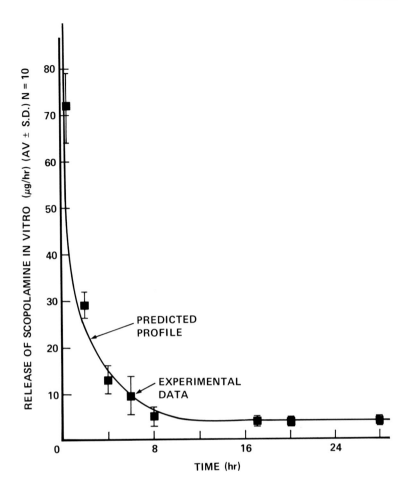

FIGURE 7. Scopolamine release rate profile (average ± SD n = 10) — comparison of theory and experiment.

the predicted mineral oil/water partition coefficients for the ionic forms would be only one to two orders of magnitude smaller than those of the corresponding free bases. Experimentally, it is observed that the mineral oil solubility of the ionic forms of these drugs is in the ppm (parts per million) range, from which partition coefficients are estimated to be three to five orders of magnitude lower than the values observed for the free bases. This suggests that for ionized forms of drugs, mineral oil does not accurately model the lipid phase of the stratum corneum. This is perhaps not unexpected, since the phospholipid bilayer, which is comprised largely of fatty zwitterion, should be able to solubilize organic electrolytes much more easily than any pure hydrocarbon or nonionic lipid.

D. Transdermal Delivery

A typical in vitro release rate time profile of scopolamine from a transdermal system into an infinite sink at isotonic and isothermal conditions is shown in Figure 7. The data points represent values experimentally measured and the solid line represents the profile predicted by theory.

For the prediction of scopolamine permeation through human skin in vivo on the basis of in vitro permeation measurements, it was assumed that the stratum corneum thickness was 40 μ and that the average steady-state diffusivity was 5×10^{-10} cm^2/sec. Using the two compartment pharmacokinetic model, the predicted urinary excretion rate profile for a

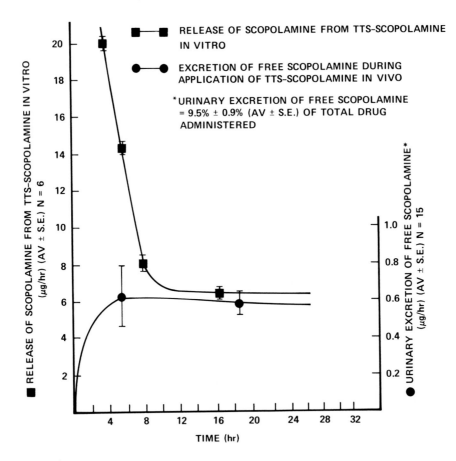

FIGURE 8.   Scopolamine excretion rate: functionality of TTS-scopolamine in vitro and in vivo.

single 24-hour application of the transdermal system is shown in Figure 8. To follow the drug input rate to the systemic circulation in vivo, the urinary excretion rate was monitored. Since only 10% of the drug is recovered in the urine in the free form following intramuscular or intravenous administration of scopolamine, it was assumed that a similar recovery would be obtained from transdermal delivery. The measured urinary excretion rates of drug following a 24-hour application of the transdermal system is also shown in Figure 8.

VI. CONCLUSIONS

The exceedingly low apparent diffusivity of most substances through the interstitial lipid phase of the stratum corneum is an anomaly of considerable note, for therein lies the origin of the remarkable impermeability of the skin. If this lipid phase were a truly homogeneous and isotropic oil, penetrant diffusion coefficients of 10^{-7} to 10^{-8} cm^2/sec (corresponding to bulk oil viscosities of 10 to 100 centipoises) would be expected.

Scheuplein's measurements of the temperature dependency of skin permeability to various substances are informative and suggestive of an explanation for the anomalous results.[1-4] Arrhenius plots of permeability vs. temperature have been used to compute activation energies for permeation, which are found to be substantially larger than expected for normal activated diffusion in liquids.

If, indeed, organized lipid bilayer membranes are largely responsible for the impermeability of stratum corneum, the lipid/protein phase partition coefficient for a particular penetrant need not be directly related to the oil/water partition coefficient of that substance, since the penetration of the permeating substance into the lipid bilayer may require alteration of its structure. Hence, compounds which may be highly lipophilic, yet which are poorly accommodated into the organized lipid phase, will display low skin permeability despite predictions to the contrary, while substances of relatively low oil affinity but which penetrate readily into and disorder the lipid microcrystalline structure may display exceedingly high skin permeability. Such substances should be able to cause marked increases in D_L, not only for themselves, but also for other concurrently permeating species.

Indeed, it seems probable that universal solvents such as dimethyl sulfoxide and hexamethyl phosphortriamide, which permeate through intact skin at phenomenally rapid rates and substantially enhance the permeation of other substances, may operate by creating controlled disorder in organized lipid membranes.

The dual mode sorption model has proved useful in the analysis of the permeation characteristics of scopolamine, through skin in vitro. The interstitial lipid phase of the tissue may be the cause for the exceedingly low apparent diffusivity of scopolamine; whereas, scopolamine sorbed by the stratum corneum is localized predominantly within the protein phase of the tissue.

The resulting insight into some of the factors that control transdermal permeation of drugs has provided a rational basis for the design and development of transdermal drug delivery systems.

ACKNOWLEDGMENT

The author wishes to gratefully acknowledge the assistance of Gail Spears, Barbara Cook, and Anna Keefover in the typing and editing of this manuscript.

REFERENCES

1. **Scheuplein, R. J.,** Mechanism of percutaneous absorption. I. Routes of penetration and the influence of solubility, *J. Invest. Dermatol,* 45, 334, 1965.
2. **Scheuplein, R. J.,** Mechanism of percutaneous absorption. II. Transient diffusion and the relative importance of various routes of skin penetration, *J. Invest. Dermatol,* 48, 79, 1967.
3. **Scheuplein, R. J. and Blank, I. H.,** Permeability of the skin, *Physiol. Rev.,* 51, 702, 1971.
4. **Scheuplein, R. J. and Blank, I. H.,** Mechanism of percutaneous absorption. IV. Penetration of nonelectrolytes (alcohols) from aqueous solutions and from pure liquids, *J. Invest. Dermatol.,* 60, 286, 1973.
5. **Michaels, A. S., Chandrasekaran, S. K., and Shaw, J. E.,** Drug permeation through human skin: theory and *in vitro* experimental measurement, *A.I.Ch.E. J.,* 21, 985, 1975.
6. **Chandrasekaran, S. K., Michaels, A. S., Campbell, P. S. and Shaw, J. E.,** Scopolamine permeation through human skin *in vitro, A.I.Ch.E. J.,* 22, 828, 1976.
7. **Chandrasekaran, S. K., Bayne, W., and Shaw, J. E.,** Pharmacokinetics of drug permeation through human skin, *J. Pharm. Sci.,* 67, 1370, 1978.

Chapter 3

PRODRUGS IN TRANSDERMAL DELIVERY*

William I. Higuchi and Cheng-Der Yu

TABLE OF CONTENTS

* A portion of this material was published in *Controlled Release Delivery Systems,* Roseman, T. J. and Mansdorf, S. Z., Marcel Dekker, New York, 1983, chap. 3.

I. INTRODUCTION

It should be timely to consider the use of prodrugs in controlled release transdermal delivery. The recent success of transdermal devices[1,2] in the market place has unveiled the high potential of transdermal delivery systems for therapeutic uses. Alza-Ciba's membrane-controlled transdermal systems for scopolamine[3-9] and nitroglycerin,[10] Searle's microsealed transdermal system,[11-15] and Key's hydrogel transdermal system[16] for nitroglycerin have successfully pioneered transdermal technology and further research is warranted for better understanding and for advancing the opportunities in this area. Transdermally delivered clonidine[17-19] (an antihypertensive) and indomethacin[20] (a nonsteroidal anti-inflammatory agent) are reportedly under development.

The use of prodrugs for improvement of drug delivery has long been of great interest to pharmaceutical scientists. One of the prevailing rationales for the use of prodrugs is to enhance drug absorption.[21-23] Another prevailing rationale is to achieve controlled release by prodrugs.[24,25] Stella[22] mentions steroids as a class of drugs where the prodrug approach has been apparently successfully utilized to promote percutaneous absorption. He supports his viewpoint by citing the acetonides of triamcinolone, fluocinolone and fluclorolone, 21-acetate of fluocinolone acetonide, valerate ester of betamethasone, propionate ester of clobetasol, pivalate and hexanoate esters of fluccortolone, acetate ester of hydrocortisone, pivalate ester of flumethasone, dipropionate ester of beclomethasone, and acetate ester of methylprednisolone as examples of topical corticosteriod esters in use. Sinkula and Yalkowsky[21] tabulated (Table 1) a list of presently marketed drugs that contain reversible linkages designed to enhance absorption of the parent molecule. Numerous examples are also given in a review by Ho et al.[23] In the area of prodrugs for achieving sustained release from intramuscular injections, a fine example may be found with the acylation of the 17 β-hydroxy group of testosterone.[26] Increasing chain length of the acyl group effectively increased the duration of action. The testosterone esters are thought to gradually leach out of an oily intramuscular depot and regenerate testosterone in the general circulation, which then exerts its androgenic activity. Other sustained release injectable steroid and other miscellaneous prodrugs are reviewed by Stella.[22] Sinkula[27] also tabulated (Table 2) a list of sustained release prodrugs.

Despite the recent success of the transdermal devices in the market place and the historical uses of steroid prodrugs, very few attempts have been made to utilize the prodrug approach in controlled release for transdermal delivery. The purpose of this chapter is to discuss rationales for prodrugs in controlled release transdermal delivery. Following a brief overview of prodrugs, a methodology is presented which combines in vitro diffusion cell experiments with freshly excised skin and theoretical techniques for describing and quantifying the transport and metabolism of prodrugs in the skin.

II. OVERVIEW OF PRODRUGS

Prodrugs have been extensively reviewed in the past. Classic reviews of Albert,[28,29] Harper,[30-32] and Ariens[33,34] were published in the 1950s and 1960s. Reviews by Stella,[22] Sinkula,[36] Sinkula and Yalkowsky,[21] and Morozowich et al.[35] were published in the 1970s. Each of these offers a different approach to the prodrug concept and readers are encouraged to refer to them. The following presents a brief overview of prodrugs.

A. Definition of Prodrug

A prodrug may be defined as a drug derivative which is converted to the drug in vivo and is able, in one or more of various possible ways, to enhance drug delivery or efficacy characteristics and, thereby, the therapeutic value of a drug. The definition may also include better patient acceptance and compliance by minimizing taste or odor problems, pain on

Table 1ᵃ

REVERSIBLE DRUG DERIVATIVES UTILIZED AS MODIFIERS OF ABSORPTION (ORAL, PERCUTANEOUS, AND PARENTERAL)

Parent molecule	Reversible modification or linkage	Route of administration	Property modified
Convallatoxin	Ketal	Oral	Resorption
Hydantoin	Alkyl ester	Oral	Absorption
	Amino ester		
Chlorphenesin	Glycine ester	Oral	Absorption
	Alanine ester		
Acetaminophen	Caffeine complex	Oral	Absorption
Acetylsalicylic acid (aspirin)	THAM salt	Oral	Absorption
	Acetamidophenyl ester	Oral	Absorption
N-Allylnoroxymorphone (naloxone)	Acetate ester	Oral	Absorption
	Sulfate ester		
Nicotinic acid	Mesoinositol pentanocotinate	Oral	Absorption
15-Methylprostaglandin $F_{2\alpha}$	Methyl ester	Oral	Absorption
Procaine	Polyethylene glycol (carbamate)	Percutaneous Conjunctival	Absorption
α-Amino-p-toluenesulfonamide (4-homosulfanilamide)	Acetate salt	Percutaneous	Absorption
Hexachlorophene	Ester	Percutaneous	Absorption
	Ether		
	Hemiester		
Oleandomycin	Acetate ester	Oral	Absorption
Erythromycin	Ester, alkyl	Oral	Absorption
Clindamycin	Ester, alkyl	Oral	Absorption
	Ester, phosphate	Intramuscular	
α-Carboxybenzylpenicillin	Ester, mono- and dialkyl	Oral	Absorption
α-Aryl-β-aminoethyl penicillin	Alkoxymethyl esters	Oral	Absorption
Penicillin, general structure	Diethylaminoethyl ester	Oral	Absorption
	Alkoxymethyl esters, ether		
α-Aminobenzylpenicillin (ampicillin)	Azide	Intravenous, oral	Absorption
6-(D-α-Sulfaminophenylacetamido) penicillin	Pivaloyloxymethyl ester	Oral	Absorption
Carbenicillin	Indanyl ester	Oral	Absorption
α-Aminobenzylpenicillin (ampicillin)	Acyloxymethyl ester	Oral	Absorption
Penicillin G Penicillin V	Amide with 1,2-benziso-thiazol-3(2H)-one 1,1-dioxide	Intramuscular	Absorption
α-Aminobenzylpenicillin (ampicillin)	N,N-Isopropylidene adduct	Oral	Absorption
Hetacillin	Pivaloyloxymethyl ester	Oral	Absorption
Doxycycline	Polymetaphosphate complex	Oral	Absorption
Colistin	Lower alkyl esters	Oral	Absorption
Tetracycline	Betaine salt	Oral	Gastric absorption
7-Acylaminocephalosporins	Ring-substituted acyloxy-benzyl esters	Oral	Absorption
	Acyloxyalkyl esters	Oral	Absorption
α-Amino (or ur-eido)cyclohexadienylalkyl penicillins and cephalosporins	Acyloxymethyl esters	Oral	Absorption

Table 1ª (continued)
REVERSIBLE DRUG DERIVATIVES UTILIZED AS MODIFIERS OF ABSORPTION (ORAL, PERCUTANEOUS, AND PARENTERAL)

Parent molecule	Reversible modification or linkage	Route of administration	Property modified
7-Acylaminocephalosporins	Imino ether	Oral	Absorption
Nandrolone	Phenylpropioate, decanoate esters	Intramuscular	Absorption
9α-Fluorohydrocortisone (fludrocortisone)	Acetate ester	Subcutaneous	Absorption
Estradiol	Enol ether Acetal	Oral, parenteral	Absorption
Oxymetholone	Ethoxycarbonate ester	Oral, subcutaneous	Absorption
Methylprednisolone	Acetate ester	Intramuscular	Absorption
Testosterone	N-Acetylglucosaminide	Oral	Absorption
	Glucosiduronate (trimethyl-silyl) ether	Oral	
19-Nortestosterone	17-β-Adamantoate	Intramuscular	Absorption
9-(β-D-Arabinofuranosyl) adenine	Acetate, formate, propionate, esters	Oral	Absorption
Cortisol, prednisolone, dexamethasone	21-Phosphate ester	Intramuscular, intravenous	Absorption
	21-Hemisuccinate ester	Subcutaneous	
Prostaglandin	Alkylsilyl ether	Percutaneous, oral, intrauterine	Absorption
Salicylic acid	Carbonate ester	Oral	Absorption

ª   Taken from Reference 21.

injection, gastrointestinal irritation, etc. The conversion to the drug may be chemical or enzymatic. Strictly speaking, the prodrug itself should not be pharmacologically active; its activity should be directly related to its ability to liberate the parent drug. However, due to the complexity of assay methodology and technique, the question of whether some prodrugs exert their effects in a derivatized form or actually require bioconversion remains largely unresolved. Steroid esters are good examples. Sinkula[37] classified this type of compound as analog-prodrug hybrid. (The term "analog" usually refers to an irreversible derivative of drug.) Table 3 is a comprehensive classification of drug modifications given by Morozowich et al.[35]

B. Applications of Prodrugs

Specific applications of prodrugs have been cited with numerous examples in Sinkula and Yalkowsky's review:[21] (1) absorption, (2) site direction, (3) depot, (4) organoleptic properties (taste and odor), and (5) irritation (intramuscular or intravenous injection and GI disturbances). Additional uses such as solving stability, solubility, or formulation problems (Figure 1) have also been reviewed by Stella[22] and Stella et al.[25] The following outlines the potential uses of prodrugs with a brief discussion and an illustrative example for each.

Oral Absorption — Ampicillin acyloxymethyl ester is a good example for the enhancement of oral absorption by prodrug approach. Ampicillin is poorly absorbed orally. Pivampicillin (pivaloyloxymethyl ester of ampicillin) was made to increase the lipophilicity and thereby the oral absorption of ampicillin. Absorption studies in humans[38] showed that peak serum levels of ampicillin from orally administered pivampicillin were more than three times greater than those from ampicillin.

Percutaneous Absorption — Many steroid esters show greater topical anti-inflammatory activity than their parent steroids. Triamcinolene acetonide, fluocinolone acetonide, and fluocinolone acetonide-21-acetate are examples of such steroid prodrugs. However, it is often questioned as to whether the steroid esters exert their activity in a derivatized form or actually require bioconversion because of the complexity of assay methodology and technique.[37]

Ophthalmic Absorption — Dipivalyl epinephrine was found to be 100 times more effective than epinephrine in the treatment of glaucoma.[39] Epinephrine, being highly polar, has difficulty in crossing the lipoidal corneal membrane. Its dipivalyl ester, being far more lipophilic than the parent compound, crosses the corneal barrier more readily and is enzymatically converted during and after transit to the target area.

Site Direction — Some recent applications of the prodrug approach have become more sophisticated. The prodrug is enzymatically converted to the active drug in the target area and therefore yields an improved therapeutic value. An example of the organ specificity is the prodrug (Pro-2-PAM) of N-methyl-pyridinium-2-carbaldoxime chloride (2-PAM-Cl).[40,41] The drug itself does not cross the blood-brain barrier. The prodrug is a tertiary amine (pKa = 6.3) of moderate lipophilicity and may easily cross the blood-brain barrier where it is oxidized to the drug (which does not cross the blood-brain barrier) and, therefore, selectively builds up in brain tissue.

Intramuscular Sustained Release or Depot — Steroids have been the subject of intense study as clinically acceptable forms of depot drugs. Testosterone palmitate and stearate have been shown to give rise to an extended duration of action and bioavailability following intramuscular injection of the esters.[42] Sinkula et al. point out that the increased duration of action is probably due to delayed absorption (solubility rate controlled) and steric hindrance (slowed hydrolysis of ester).

Taste Masking — Chloramphenicol palmitate[43] is a well-known example. Clindamycin-2-palmitate[44] was also found to be devoid of the bitter taste.

Gastrointestinal Irritation — Salicylic acid is known to cause gastrointestinal irritation. The hexylcarbonate ester of salicylic acid was found to cause far less gastrointestinal irritation in animal studies.[45] It is thought that the carbonate ester is more lipophilic and therefore allows absorption and distribution over a greater area of the gastrointestinal tract, thus reducing localized irritation.

Injection Site Irritation — Clindamycin-2-phosphate is a fine example of a prodrug with decreased pain on intramuscular injection.[46] Morozowich et al.[35] noted the underlying mechanism and the rationale for the phosphate prodrug as follows: lincomycin produces little pain on intramuscular injection whereas clindamycin produces an intense pain response. The 40-fold greater partition coefficient of clindamycin over lincomycin presumably permits increased local cell penetration resulting in pain, and a polar derivative such as the phosphate was proposed as a solution to the problem. Clindamycin-2-phosphate showed little local irritation and pain on injection.

Chemical Stability — In an attempt to improve the solid-state stability of dinoprostone (an E type prostaglandin), Morozowich et al.[47] synthesized various parasubstituted phenyl esters of this drug. The crystalline esters were shown to have improved solid-state stability over the parent compound. The improved solid-state stability was attributed to the stabilization by the crystal lattice.[47]

Aqueous Solubility — Chloramphenicol has an aqueous solubility of 2.5 mg/mℓ. The monosodium salt of chloramphenicol hemi-sussinate, being appreciably more water soluble, has made the intravenous or intramuscular injection possible (dose range is around 25 to 30 mg/kg).

C. Pro-Moieties of Prodrugs and Their Enzyme Specificity

The most frequently modified functional groups of drug molecules in prodrug design are

Table 2ª
CLINICALLY USEFUL CHEMICAL SUSTAINED RELEASE PREPARATIONS

Parent molecule	Chemical extender	Trade (generic) name	Approximate duration of therapeutic activity	Route of administration	Use
9-fluoro-16 hydroxyprednisolone	Acetonide	Triamcinolone Hexacetonide	3—4 weeks	Intraarticular	Antiinflammatory
Methylprednisolone	Acetate ester	Depo-Medrol	1—7 days	Intramuscular	Antiinflammatory
Testosterone	Cyclopentylpropionate ester	Depo-Testosterone	2—4 weeks	Intramuscular	Androgenic steroid
	Heptanoate ester	Delatestryl	2—4 weeks	Intramuscular	Androgenic steroid
19-Nortestosterone	Phenylpropionate ester	Durabolin	1 week	Intramuscular	Anabolic steroid
	Decanoate ester	Deca-Durabolin	3—4 weeks	Intramuscular	Anabolic steroid
Estradiol + testosterone	Cyclopentylpropionate esters	Depo-Testadiol	3—4 weeks	Intramuscular	Androgen/esterogen
	Valerate esters	Deladumone	1—3 weeks	Intramuscular	Androgen/estrogen
Estradiol	Benzoate ester	Estradiol benzoate	1—2 days	Intramuscular	Estrogenic steroid
	Cyclopentylpropionate ester	Depo-Estradiol Cypionate	1 week	Intramuscular	Estrogenic steroid
	Phosphate ester	Polyestradiol phosphate	2—4 weeks	Intramuscular	Prostatic carcinoma
Hydroxyprogesterone	Caproate ester	Delautin	9—17 days	Intramuscular	Progestin
Desoxycorticosterone	Pivalate ester	Percorten Pivalate	4 weeks	Intramuscular	Adrenocortical insufficiency
	Acetate ester	Percorten acetate	8—12 months	Subcutaneous implant	Adrenocortical insufficiency
Dexamethasone	Acetate ester	Decadron-LA	1—3 weeks	Intramuscular	Antiinflammatory
Medroxyprogesterone	Acetate ester	Depo-Provera	3 months	Intramuscular	Endometriosis
			1—4 weeks		Endometrial carcinoma
			3 months +		Contraception
Dextroamphetamine	Tannate salt	Obotan	1 day	Oral	Appetite suppressant
Penicilliin G	Procaine salt	Duracillin A.S.	1 day	Intramuscular	Antibacterial
	Benzathine salt	Bicillin LA	1—2 days	Intramuscular	Antibacterial
Epinephrine	Dipivalate ester	Dipivefrin	12 hours	Intraocular	Antiglaucoma agent

Fluphenazine	Heptanoate ester	Prolixin enanthate	2—4 weeks	Intramuscular	Antipsychotic
	Decanoate ester	Prolixin decanoate	2—4 weeks	Intramuscular	Antipsychotic
Perphenazine	Heptanoate ester	Cetrane	4 weeks	Intramuscular	Antipsychotic
Pipothiazine	Undecylenate ester		2 weeks	Intramuscular	Antipsychotic
	Palmitate ester	Piportil	4 weeks	Intramuscular	Antipsychotic
Flupenthixol	Decanoate ester	Depixol	2—3 weeks	Intramuscular	Antipsychotic
Sulfadiazine	Silver salt	Silvadene	24 hr	Topical	Anti-infective
Insulin	Zinc suspension	Semilente iletin	12—16 hr	Subcutaneous	Insulin preparation
	Zinc suspension	Ultralente iletin	>36 hr	Subcutaneous	Insulin preparation

[a] Taken from Reference 27.

Table 3[a]
CLASSIFICATION OF DRUG MODIFICATION

Term	Type of Modification	Biologically Active Species	General Utility
Analog	Structural modification or substitutent group synthesis	Active per se	Improve potency and specificity

$$Cl \text{---} \bigcirc \text{---} CH_2\text{--}CH(OH)\text{--}CH_2\text{--}OH$$

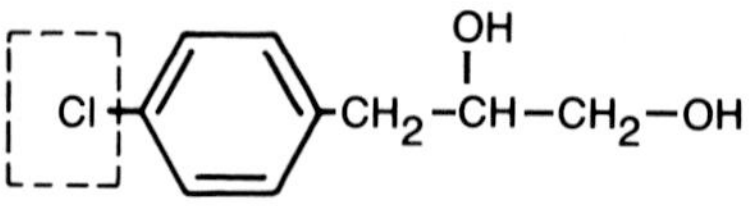

Chlorophenesin

| Prodrug Derivative prodrug | Functional group derivative | Cleaved in vivo to active parent drug | Improve biopharmaceutical properties |

$$NO_2\text{---}\bigcirc\text{---}CH(OH)\text{--}CH(NH\text{--}C(=O)\text{--}CHCl_2)\text{--}CH_2\text{--}O\text{--}C(=O)\text{--}C_{15}H_{31}$$

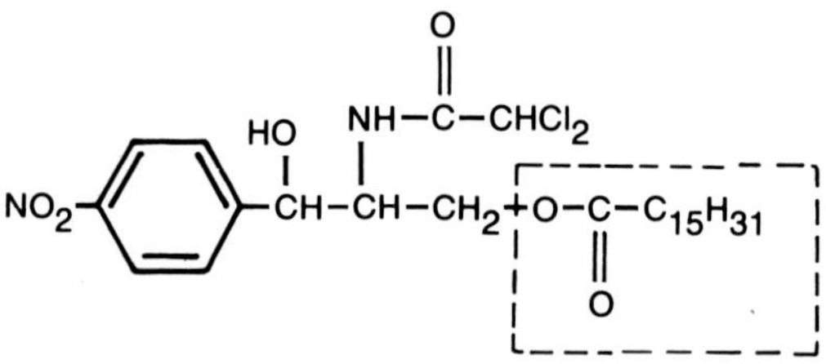

Chloramphenicol Palmitate

| Analog prodrug | Structural modification or substituent synthesis | Metabolically transformed to active drug in vivo | Improve biopharmaceutical properties |

$$\text{Griseofulvin structure: } CH_3O,\ OCH_3,\ CH_3O,\ Cl,\ OH$$

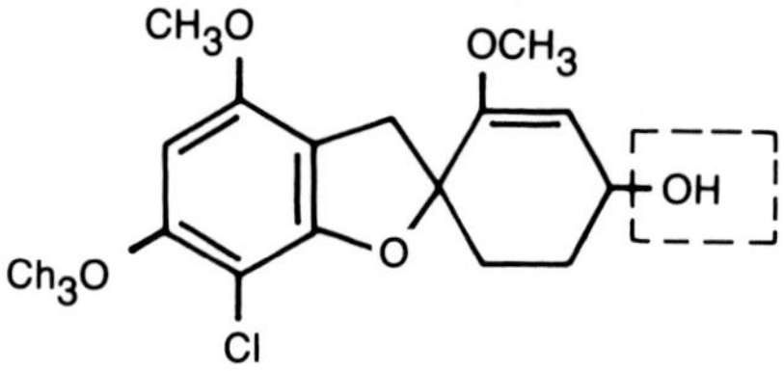

Griseofulvin Alcohol

| Derivative | Functional group derivative | Active per se | Improve potency and specificity and/or biopharmaceutical properties |

$$Cl\text{---}\bigcirc\text{---}O\text{--}CH_2\text{--}CH(OH)\text{--}CH_2\text{--}O\text{--}C(=O)\text{--}NH_2$$

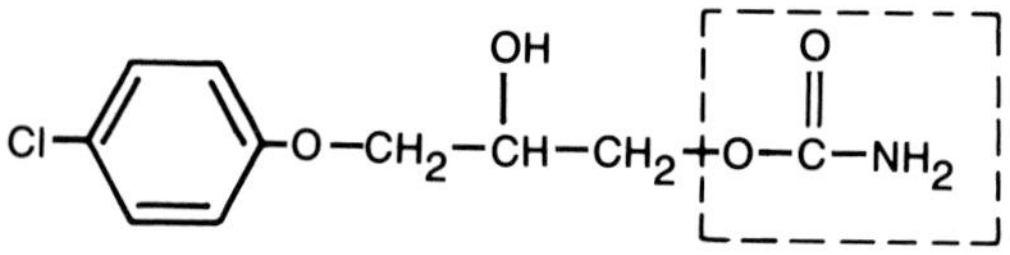

Chlorphenesin Carbamate

[a]   Taken from Reference 35.

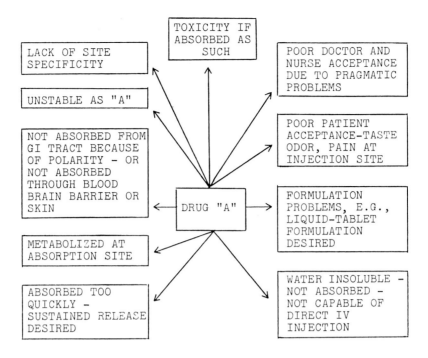

FIGURE 1.   Problems which can be solved by prodrug approach.[22]

the carboxyl, hydroxyl, and amino groups. The carboxyl group can be modified into esters or amides; the hydroxyl group can be modified into acyl esters, hemiesters, carbonate esters, phosphate esters, nitrate esters, acetals, ketals, and ethers; the amino group can be modified into amides, peptides, and carbamates. In the following, examples of each of the three categories will be given and their enzymatic conversions briefly discussed with the intent of presenting an introductory overview of the subject. Comprehensive reviews can be found in the articles by Sinkula,[36] Sinkula et al.,[21] Morozowich et al.,[35] Amidon et al.,[48] Stella,[22] and Stella et al.[25]

1. Derivatives of Carboxylic Acid-Containing Drugs

Ester formation between an alcohol and a carboxylic acid group of the parent compound is one of the most frequently used approaches in prodrug design. A few examples are given in Table 4. The resultant esters can be hydrolyzed by nonspecific or specific esterases. Krisch[49] gives an excellent review on enzymology of carboxylic ester hydrolases. Amidon et al.[48] reviewed carboxylic ester hydrolases and lipases with emphasis on prodrug considerations. Sinkula et al.[21] have comprehensively reviewed esterases and phosphatases. Morozowich et al.[35] discussed substituent effects on enzymatic specificity for prodrugs. Table 5 lists examples of enzyme substrates for esterases. Table 6 tabulates host tissues in which esterases and other enzymes can be found.

a. Aliphatic, Aromatic, and Thioalkyl Esters

Aspirin is a carboxylic acid-containing drug for which many prodrugs have been made to solve various problems associated with the compound. The acetamidophenyl ester (I) of aspirin was shown to cause fewer incidences of gastrointestinal tract bleeding.[50] The (1'-ethoxy) ethyl ester (IV) of aspirin (see Table 4) was shown to be less irritating to the gastrointestinal tract.[52] The aromatic esters and activated esters such as compound IV are rapidly hydrolyzed by esterases. Nonspecific esterases hydrolyze a variety of ester types including aliphatic, aromatic and thio-esters, and a number of aromatic amides.[49] Rapid

Table 4
PRODRUGS OF CARBOXYL GROUP-CONTAINING COMPOUNDS

Parent Drug	Prodrug	Improvement	Ref.
Aspirin, R = H 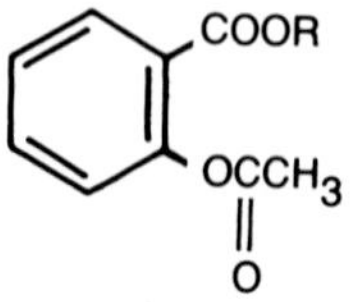	Acetamidophenyl ester 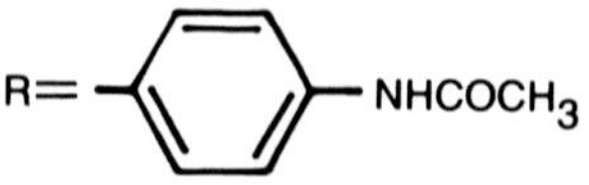	GI irritation	50
	Methylthiomethyl ester	Percutaneous absorption	51
	R = –CH$_2$SCH$_3$		
	Methylsulfinylmethyl ester	Percutaneous absorption	51
	R = –CH$_2$SOCH$_3$		
	(1′-Ethoxy)ethyl ester	GI irritation	52
	α-D-1-2-deoxyglucopyranosyl ester 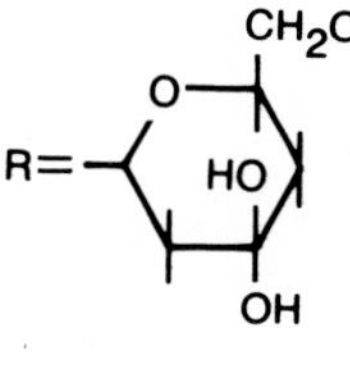	GI irritation	53, 54
Dinoprostone, R = H	p-Substituted phenyl esters	Chemical stability	47
	R′ = various substitution. See Ref. 55		
	Alkyl esters	Duration of activity	55, 56
	R = various chain length. See Ref. 56		
Clofibric acid, R = H 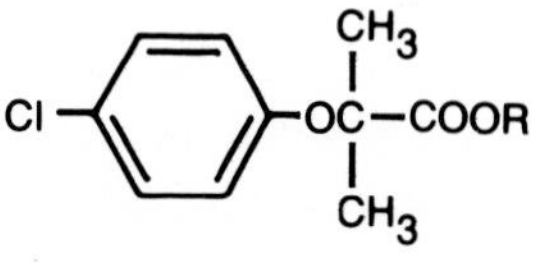	Clofibrate	Oral absorption	57, 58
	R = CH$_2$CH$_3$		

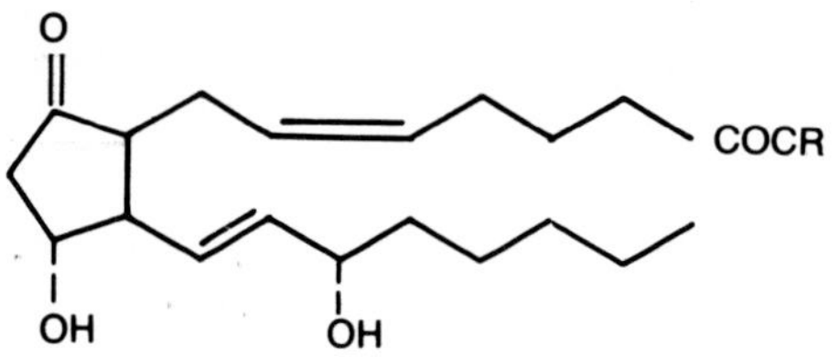

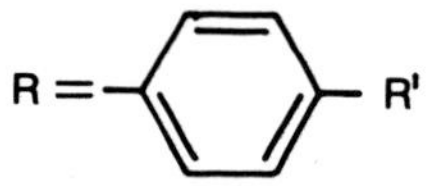

Aspirin structure:
COOR
OCCH$_3$ (=O)

R= (phenyl)–NHCOCH$_3$

α-D-1-2-deoxyglucopyranosyl ester:
CH$_2$OH, HO, OH, V

Dinoprostone structure with COCR

R = (phenyl) R′ VI

Clofibric acid structure:
Cl–(phenyl)–OC(CH$_3$)(CH$_3$)–COOR

Table 4 (Continued)
PRODRUGS OF CARBOXYL GROUP-CONTAINING COMPOUNDS

Parent Drug	Prodrug	Improvement	Ref.
Ampicillin, R = H	Pivampicillin	Oral absorption	60

$$R = CH_2-O-\overset{O}{\overset{\|}{C}}-\overset{CH_3}{\overset{\|}{C}}-CH_3$$
$$\underset{CH_3}{}$$

| | Bacampicillin | Oral absorption | 61 |

$$R = \overset{CH_3}{\overset{\|}{CH}}-O-\overset{O}{\overset{\|}{C}}-O-CH_2-CH_3$$

| | Talampicillin | Oral absorption | 62 |

$$R = CH \overset{O}{\diagup} C = O$$

| Carbenicillin, R = R′ = H | Indanyl ester | Acid stability Oral absorption | 63 |

$$R = $$

$$R = Na$$

| Phenoxymethylpenicillin, R = OH | Saccharimide | Oral absorption | 64 |

$$R = -N\overset{SO_2}{\diagup}\overset{}{\diagdown}\overset{C}{\overset{\|}{O}}$$

| Penicillin G, R = OH | Amide | IM absorption | 59 |

$$R = NH_2$$

Table 5ᵃ
EXAMPLES OF ESTERASE SUBSTRATES

Carboxyl esters
  Esters of unsubstituted fatty acids
    Phenyl formate (acetate, propionate, butyrate, valerate)
    Ethyl formate (acetate, propionate, valerate)
    M-Carboxyphenyl esters of a homologous series of n-fatty acids (chain length from C_2 to C_{12})
    Ethyl acetate
    Glyceryl triacetate (triacetin)
    p-Nitrophenyl acetate
    o-Nitrophenyl acetate
    2,6-Dichlorobenzenone-indophenyl acetate
    Vitamin A acetate
    Methyl butyrate
    Methyl butyrate (3-methylbutyrate, pentanoate, 3- and 4-methylpentanoate, hexanoate, heptanoate)
    Glyceryl tributyrate (tributyrin)
    Ethyl butyrate
    O-, m-,and p-Nitrophenyl butyrate
    2,4-Dinitrophenyl butyrate
    m-(n-Pentanoyloxy) benzoic acid
    m-(n-Heptanoyloxy) benzoic acid
  Esters of other acids
    Ethyl benzoate (benzenesulfonate, lactate, acetoacetate; diethyl succinate, fumarate, asparate; p-hydroxy-
       benzoate, bromomalonate, terephthalate, and other ethyl esters)
    Procaine (2-diethylaminoethyl p-aminbenzoate)
    L-Tyrosine ethyl ester (and many other amino acid esters)
Thioesters
  6-S- and 8-S-Acetoacetyl monothioloctanoate
  8-S-acetoacetyl, 6-ethyl monothioloctanoate
  8-S-acetoacetyl dihydrolipoic acid
  6-S- and 8-S-acetyl dihydrolipoic acid
  S-acetyl- and S-acetoacetyl-BAL
  p-Nitrothiophenyl hippurate
  Thiophenyl acetate
Aromatic amides
  Acetanilide
  Phenacetin
  Monethylglycine 2,6-xylidide
  Diethylglycine 2,6-xylidide (xylocaine; lidocaine)
  N-(n-Butylamino) acetyl 2-chloro, 6-methylanilide · HCl (Hostacaine; butacetloid)
  L-Leucyl p-nitroanilide
  L-Leucyl β-naphthylamide
  2-(N-4-n-Propylaminoacetyl)-sulfanilamido 4,6-dimethylpyridine HCl

ᵃ   Taken from Reference 49. See original article for references.

hydrolysis of compound IV also occurs in water to give aspirin. At pH = 3.2 (25°C), the $t_{1/2}$ for hydrolysis is 3.2 sec and the reaction is pH dependent.[52] The labile nature of the ester is expected to facilitate in vivo cleavage. Another acylal derivative, α-D-2-deoxyglu-copyranosyl ester (V)[53] of aspirin, was shown to hydrolyze to aspirin in vitro with a halflife of 7 min at 37°C.[54]

Thioalkyl esters of aspirin were investigated for improvement in percutaneous absorption.[51] The methylthiomethyl ester (II) and the methylsulfinylmethyl ester (III) of aspirin were found to penetrate freshly excised hairless mice skin rather easily with the simultaneous hydrolysis of the two esters. However, contrary to in vivo observations in dogs, where significant amounts of aspirin were found to form, the prodrugs cleaved to salicylic acid and/or salicylate esters rather than to aspirin.

Morozowich et al.[47] synthesized a series of p-substituted phenyl esters (VI) of dinoprostone

Table 6[a]
REVERSIBLE DERIVATIVE AND PRODRUG LINKAGES AND THEIR HYDROLYZING ENZYMES

Linkage	Hydrolyzing enzyme	Tissue
Ester		
Short and medium-chain aliphatic	Cholinesterase	Liver, kidney, gut
	Ester hydrolase	Blood, intestinal mucosa
	Lipase	
	Cholesterol esterase	
	Acetylcholinesterase	
	Acetyl esterase	
	Aldehyde oxidase	General distribution
	Lipase	Liver
	Carboxypeptidase	Gut
Long-chain aliphatic	Pancreatic lipase	
Carbonate	Pancreatin	Intestine
	Lipase	
	Aliesterase	
	Carboxypeptidase	
	Cholinesterase	Blood
Hemiester	Esterases	Blood
Phosphate, organic	Acid phosphatase	Blood
	Alkaline phosphatase	Blood
	Acid phosphatase III	Blood
Pyrophosphate	Pyrophosphatase I	Liver, gut, blood
Sulfate, organic	Steroid sulfatase	Liver, blood
	Arylsulfohydrolase A and B (phenolsulfatase, arylsulfatase)	Liver
	Arylsulfohydrolase C	Liver
	Estrogen sulfohydrolase	Liver, gut
	Steroid-3β-sulfohydrolase	Liver
	Steroid-21-sulfatase	Placenta
Amide	Amidase	Liver
		Neoplastic tissue
		Walker carcinosarcoma 256
		Dunning rat leukemia
		Neoplastic tissue
Amino acid	Proteolytic enzymes	Gut
		Neoplastic tissue
	Chymotrypsins A and B	
	Trypsin	
	Carboxypeptidase A	
	Carboxypeptidase B	
Azo	Azoreductase	Liver
		Walker rat carcinoma
		Sarcoma 180
		Adenocarcinoma 755
		Lymphoid leukemia L-1210
		Liver
		Gut microflora
Carbamate	Carbamidase	Liver
		Walker carcinosarcoma 256 (rats)
		Adenocarcinoma 755 (mice)
		Liver
Phosphamide	Phosphoramidases	Neoplastic tissue (liver)
		Liver

Table 6ᵃ (Continued)
REVERSIBLE DERIVATIVE AND PRODRUG LINKAGES AND THEIR
HYDROLYZING ENZYMES

Linkage	Hydrolyzing enzyme	Tissue
Glucosiduronate (β-glucuronide)	β-Glucuronidase	Liver Gut Blood Gut microflora
N-Acetylglucosaminide	α-N-Acetylglucosaminidase β-N-Acetylglucosaminidase	Liver, gut, blood
β-Glucoside	β-Glucosidase	Gut, liver Gut, microflora

ᵃ   Taken from Reference 21.

(a prostaglandin E_2) and showed an improved solid-state stability of these crystalline esters over the parent compound. Several of these esters showed activities comparable to the parent compound. Alkyl esters of dinoprostone were also made in an attempt to prolong the duration of activity of the parent compound.[55,56] The greater potency found for these esters has been attributed to a lengthening of the metabolic half-life of the ester form relative to the parent acid prostaglandin.

Clofibrate (VII) is a simple ester prodrug with excellent oral efficacy. The ester hydrolyzes rapidly in vivo to clofibric acid which was shown to be the active species.[57,58]

Penicillin esters are fine examples of activated ester prodrugs. Simple aliphatic esters of penicillins are not active in vivo in higher animals[59] likely due to high steric hindrance of the carboxyl group. Pivampicillin (VIII),[60] bacampicillin (IX),[61] and Talampicillin (IX)[62] all contain activated acyloxymethyl group. Pivampicillin hydrolyzes readily in vivo to give the ampicillin ester of hydroxy methanol. The latter is unstable and spontaneously cleaves to ampicillin and formaldehyde. Likewise, bacampicillin and talampicillin cleave to give ampicillin and acetaldehyde and α-carboxybenzaldehyde.

Acid stability is one of the major advantages of carbencillin esters. Carbenicillin indanyl sodium (XI) showed no loss of activity while disodium carbenicillin lost 99.2% of its antibacterial activity after incubating in synthetic gastric juice at 37°C for 1 hr.[65] The indanyl ester was shown to be rapidly and completely absorbed from the G.I. tract with subsequent hydrolysis to carbencillin by nonspecific serum and tissue esterases.[63]

b. Amides

Phenoxymethylpenicillin saccharimide (XII) is an orally active penicillin amide prodrug.[64] The activity is attributed to the highly activated nature of the amide bond. Simple amines of penicillins have little activity, likely due to the steric hindrance of the carboxyl group. The amide of penicillin G (XIII) has approximately 10% of the activity of penicillin G.[59]

2. Derivatives of Hydroxyl Group-Containing Drugs

The hydroxyl group is the most versatile functional group for chemical modifications. It can be modified into an acyl ester, hemiester, phosphate ester, carbonate ester, nitrate ester, alkyl ether, silyl ether, and acetal derivatives. Table 7 lists a few examples for each of the chemical modifications.

a. Acyl Esters

Chloramphenicol has two hydroxyl groups which can be modified. The terminal hydroxyl group, being less sterically hindered is commonly used for prodrug modification. Chlor-

Table 7
DERIVATIVES OF HYDROXYL GROUP-CONTAINING COMPOUNDS

Parent Drug	Prodrug	Improvement	Ref.
Chloramphenicol, R = H	Palmitate ester	Taste	43

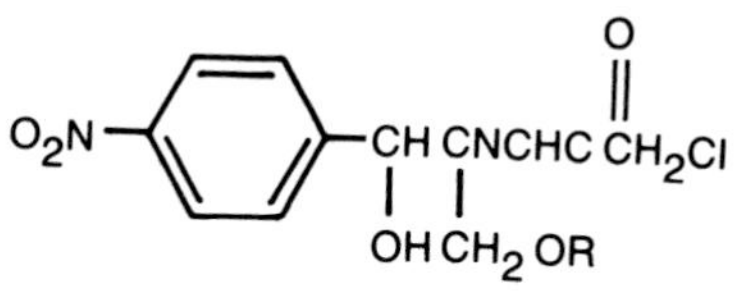

$$R = -\overset{\displaystyle O}{\overset{\displaystyle \|}{C}}(CH_2)_{14}CH_3$$

| | Succininate hemi-ester | Solubility | 66—69 |

$$R = -\overset{\displaystyle O}{\overset{\displaystyle \|}{C}}(CH_2)_2COONa$$

Irritation on injection

| Clindamycin, R = H | 2-Acyl ester | Taste | 44 |

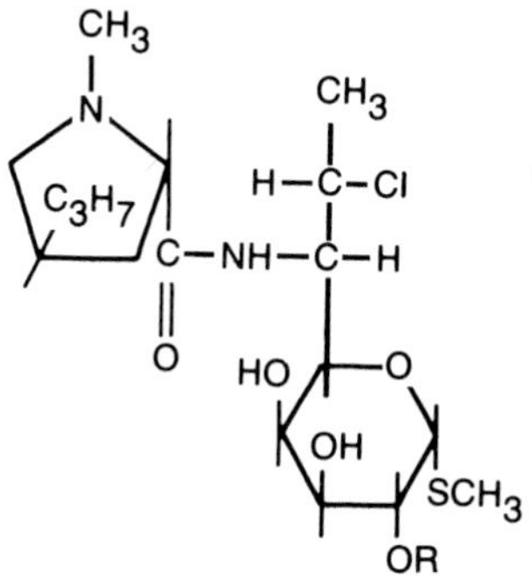

$$R = -\overset{\displaystyle O}{\overset{\displaystyle \|}{C}}(CH_2)_nCH_3$$

n = Various chain length
See Ref. 44

| | 2-Phosphate ester | Solubility | 65, 70 |

$$R = -\overset{\displaystyle OH}{\overset{\displaystyle |}{\underset{\displaystyle \underset{O}{\|}}{P}}}-OH$$

Irritation on injection   46

| | 2-Alkylcarbonate ester | Taste | 44 |

$$R = -\overset{\displaystyle O}{\overset{\displaystyle \|}{C}}O(CH_2)_nCH_3$$

n = Various chain length
See Ref. 44

Table 7 (Continued)
DERIVATIVES OF HYDROXYL GROUP-CONTAINING COMPOUNDS

Parent Drug	Prodrug	Improvement	Ref.
Lincomycin, R = R′ = H	7-Acyl esters	Taste	71, 72

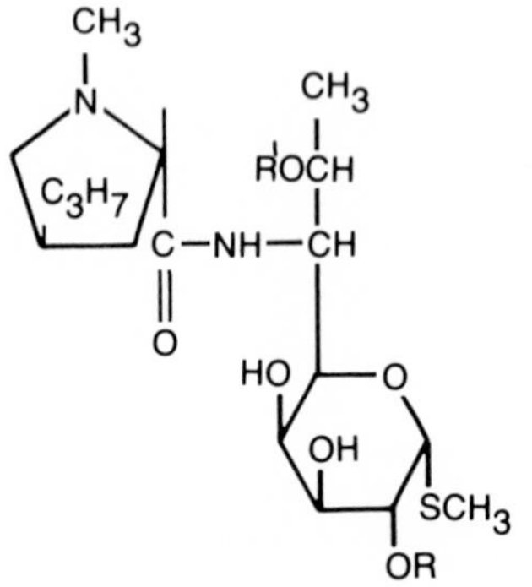

R = H

R′ = –CR″
$\quad\quad$‖
$\quad\quad$O

R″ = Various acyl group;
See Ref. 71

| | 2-Phosphate | Taste | 73 |

$$R = -\underset{\underset{O}{\|}}{\overset{\overset{OH}{|}}{P}}-OH$$

| Salicylic acid, R = H | Carbonate ester | GI irritation | 45, 74 |

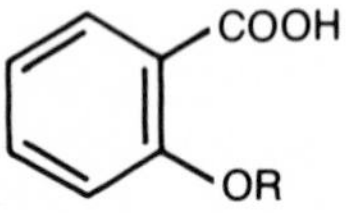

$$R = -\underset{\underset{O}{\|}}{C}OR'$$

R′ = ethyl, n-butyl, n-
hexyl, or trichloroethyl

| Pentaerythritol trinitrate, R = H 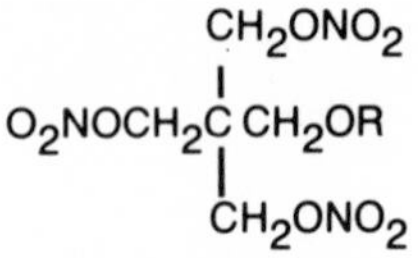 | Pentaerythritol tetranitrate | Duration of activity | 75 |

CH_2ONO_2
|
$O_2NOCH_2C\ CH_2OR$
|
CH_2ONO_2

R = –NO$_2$

| Acetaminophen, R = H 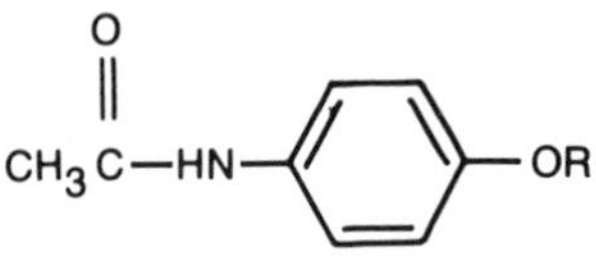 | 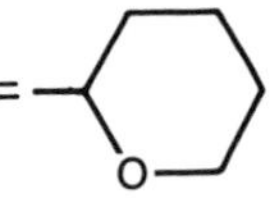 Tetrahydropyranyl ether | Duration of activity | 78 |

$$CH_3\underset{\overset{\|}{O}}{C}-HN-\!\!\!\bigcirc\!\!\!-OR$$

R=

Table 7 (Continued)
DERIVATIVES OF HYDROXYL GROUP-CONTAINING COMPOUNDS

Parent Drug	Prodrug	Improvement	Ref.
Allopurinol, R = H	Ethoxyethylidenyl	Dissolution	79

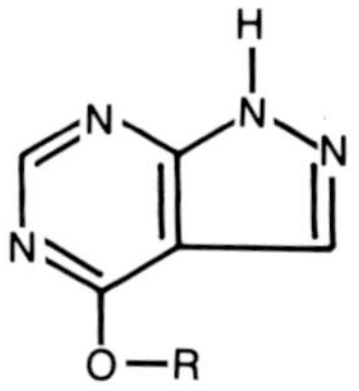

$$R = -CH-O-CH_2CH_3$$ (with CH_3 on the CH)

	Tetrahydropyranyl ether 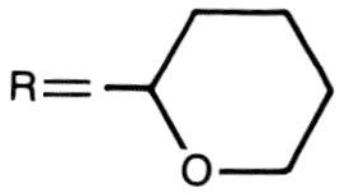	Dissolution	79

R=

Ethynylestradiol, R = H 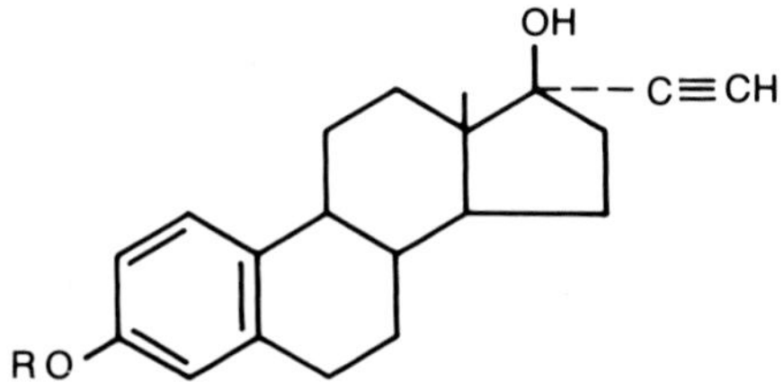	3-Cyclopentyl ether 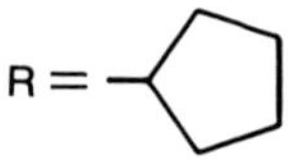	Duration of activity	80

R=

Methylephedrine, R = H	Silyl ethers	Duration of activity	81

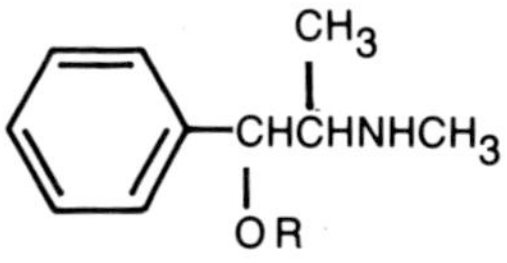

$$R = -Si-R'$$ (with R' above and below)

R = various alkyl group
See Ref. 81

Nicotinaldehyde 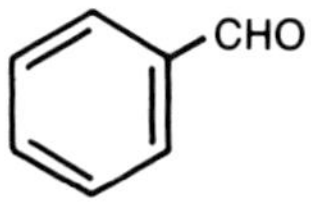	Acetal 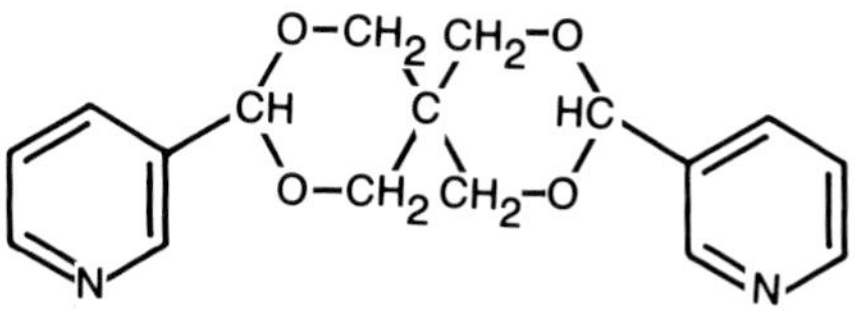	Duration of activity	82

amphenicol palmitate (XIV) is less bitter than its parent compound because of its low solubility.[43] The ester is well absorbed orally and cleaves to give chloramphenicol in vivo readily by serum and tissue esterases. The succinate hemi-ester of chloramphenicol (XV) was made to increase the aqueous solubility of chloramphenicol and thereby make the injectable route possible.[66-69]

b. Phosphate Esters

Clindamycin is another antibiotic which gives an unpleasant bitter taste. Various acyl esters (XVI) and carbonate esters (XVII) of clindamycin were made to reduce the bitter taste of the parent compound.[44] For the injectable form, phosphate ester (XVII) was made to increase the solubility as well as to ease the pain on injection.[46,65,70] Phosphate esters are readily hydrolyzed in vivo by the widely distributed phosphatase enzymes. Interestingly, phosphate esters show excellent aqueous solution stability in the di-anionic form (at a pH of around 7) and some phosphates are stable for 1 to 2 years in aqueous solutions.[71] Few acylesters can achieve comparable solution stability.

Lincomycin 7-acyl esters (XVIII)[72] and the 2-phosphate (XIX)[73] have been synthesized as prodrugs of lincomycin.

c. Carbonate Esters

Alkylcarbonate esters (XX) of salicylic acid exhibit a greatly reduced incidence of gastric irritation compared to aspirin.[45] The carbonate esters are readily hydrolyzed in vivo.[74]

d. Nitrate Esters

Pentaerythritol tetranitrate (XXI) is metabolized in humans to pentaerythritol trinitrate and possesses a greater vasodilator activity than the parent compound.[75] The transformation from the tetra- to the trinitrate occurs primarily in the liver and is catalyzed by the enzyme glutathione-organic nitrate reductase.[76] Various aspects of nitrate ester metabolism have been reviewed.[77]

e. Alkyl Ethers

Most of the ethers employed as prodrugs consist of acid labile ethers. Tetrahydropyranyl ethers of acetaminophen (XXII) and allopurinol (XXIV) are examples of the acid labile ethers. Compound XXII was reported to hydrolyze to the parent compound with a half-life of approximately 10 sec at pH 1.1 (25°C).[78] Compound XXIV has a half-life of 12 min in 0.1 N HCl at 37°C.[79] The ethoxyethylidenyl ether (XXIII) of allopurinol is also acid labile with a $t_{1/2}$ of 7.7 min in 0.1 N HCl at 37°C.[79]

Ethynylestradiol-3-cyclopentyl ether (XXV), an acid stable ether, has been used to prolong the steroid activity. The mechanism for the prolongation of activity was shown to be the uptake of compound XXV by fatty tissues in the body. When given orally, compound XXV is found largely in the fatty tissues for periods in excess of 72 hr.[80] However, whether this compound is a prodrug has not been established.

f. Silyl Ethers

The silyl ether of methylephedrine (XXVI) significantly improves the lipophilicity of the parent drug and thereby enhances its activity.[81] Silyl ethers are rapidly hydrolyzed in water.

g. Acetals

The acetal of nicotinaldehyde (XXVII) is an impressive example of achieving chemical sustained release by prodrug formation. A comparison of the blood levels of nicotinic acid following the administration of nicotinic acid alone and compound XXVII showed a remarkable sustained release effect for compound XXVII.[82] Nicotinic acid alone gave a level of 69 μg/mℓ at 1 hr with a drop to zero at 6 hr. Compound XXVII gave maximum levels of the intact derivative at 6 hr and the levels slowly declined thereafter. The levels of nicotinic acid resulting from compound XXVII is low but sustained with levels of around 1.0 μg/mℓ up to 44 hr. Formation of nicotinic acid from the derivative occurs via a sequential process involving cleavage of the acetal followed by oxidation of nicotinaldehyde to nicotinic acid.

3. Derivatives of Amino Group-Containing Drugs

Amino group-containing drugs can be modified into amide, carbamate, azo, or peptide prodrugs. Examples are listed in Table 8.

Azo Derivatives — Prontosil (XXVIII) is a unique azo type prodrug of sulfanilamide.[83] The enzyme involved with converting compound XXVIII to sulfamilamide is azo reductase. The enzyme is present in the gastrointestinal tract and liver.

Amides — The *N*-acetyl amide of sulfisoxazole (XXIX)[84] has a reduced bitter taste compared to its parent drug. The *N*-acetyl amide group is an activated amide which is readily hydrolyzed in vivo.

Carbamates — The *O*-nitrophenyl carbamate of amphetamine (XXX)[85] is an example of a carbamate prodrug. Compound XXX was shown to enter mouse brain rapidly and readily hydrolyze subsequently.[85] The hydrolysis of carbamates is catalyzed by nonspecific amidases and esterases.

Peptides — Compound XXXI was shown to be an orally active peptidyl prodrug of aracytidine.[86] The peptide linkage is cleaved in vivo by pepidases. These enzymes are present in duodenal and intestinal epithelia.

III. RATIONALE FOR PRODRUGS IN TRANSDERMAL DELIVERY

A drug must reach the "target site" before its pharmacological response can be elicited. There are barriers that might limit the ability of a drug to reach its "target site". In the case of a transdermally delivered drug, two major barriers may be encountered: a physicochemical barrier, skin permeability, and a biological barrier such as enzymatic degradation. Prodrugs may be used to increase skin permeability and/or to alter metabolism of the drug.

A. Physicochemical Considerations

Permeation of drug substances through the skin may be illustrated by Figure 2 (a and b). The figures depict drug concentration gradients across various strata of the skin during steady-state diffusion. For a polar compound, the gradient across the stratum corneum may be greater than those across the epidermis and dermis since the stratum corneum is usually the predominant barrier. However, for a nonpolar compound, the diffusional resistances of the epidermis and the dermis could become rate limiting. Regardless for a polar or nonpolar compound, the general phenomenon of skin permeation can be described by the Fick's diffusion law as follows:

$$J_i = \frac{D_i(C_{i-1} - C_i)}{h_i} \tag{1}$$

where J_i is the steady-state flux across the ith stratum of the skin, D_i is the diffusivity of the drug in the ith stratum, C_{i-1} and C_i are the drug concentrations at the influx side interface and the efflux side interface of the ith stratum, and h_i is the thickness of the ith stratum.

The partition coefficient (K) is also a very important factor which affects the transdermal delivery of a drug. As illustrated by Figure 2 (a and b), the drug concentration at the inner

Table 8
PRODRUGS OF AMINO GROUP-CONTAINING COMPOUNDS

Parent Drug	Prodrug	Improvement	Ref.
Sulfanilamide	Prontosil		83

H_2NSO_2—⬡—NH_2

H_2NSO_2—⬡—$N{=}N$—⬡(H_2N)—NH_2

| Sulfisoxazole, R = H | N-acetyl amide | Taste | 84 |

H_2N—⬡—SO_2—$N(R)$—C(—N═, —CH$_3$, O—, —CH$_3$ oxazole)

$$R = -\overset{\displaystyle \|}{\underset{\displaystyle O}{C}}CH_3$$

| Amphetamine, R = H | Carbamate | Duration of activity | 85 |

⬡—CH_2—$\overset{CH_3}{CH}$—NHR

$$R = -\overset{O}{\overset{\|}{C}}-O-\text{(o-}NO_2\text{-phenyl)}$$

| ara-Cytidine, R = R′ = H | Peptidyl derivative | Oral absorption | 86 |
| | N⁴-tert-butoxycarbonyl-glycyl-L-arginyl) | | |

(cytidine structure with NHR, O═, N, N ring; R′OH$_2$C, HO, HO on sugar)

$$R = -\overset{O}{\overset{\|}{C}}CHNH\overset{O}{\overset{\|}{C}}CH_2NH\overset{O}{\overset{\|}{C}}O(CH_2)_3CH_3$$

$$\underset{(CH_2)_3NHC NH_2}{|}$$
$$\underset{NH}{\overset{\|}{}}$$

R′ = H or palmityl, benzoly, adamantoyl

FOR POLAR SOLUTES: $P_{SC} \ll P_E$ OR P_D

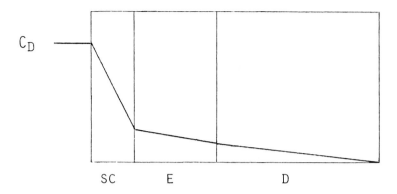

FOR NONPOLAR SOLUTES: $P_{SC} \gg P_E$ OR P_D

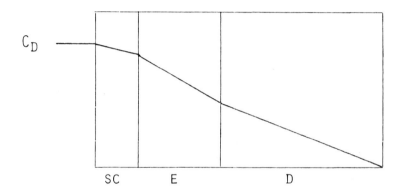

FIGURE 2.   Drug concentration gradients across stratum corneum (SC), epidermis (E), and dermis (D) at steady-state.

surface of the stratum corneum is not usually equal to that in the external phase but is related to it in accord with the partition coefficient. For a polar compound applied to the skin in a aqueous solution, the concentration at the inner surface of the stratum corneum is reduced to that in the external phase. On the other hand, for a nonpolar compound, the concentration at the inner surface of the stratum corneum is increased to K times of that in the external phase. To best illustrate the effect of the partition coefficient, consider first the case of a single laminate membrane separating two chambers of a diffusion cell with the same solvent on both sides. The flux for this situation is given by:

$$J = \frac{K \, D \, \Delta C}{h} \tag{2}$$

or

$$J = P \, \Delta C \tag{3}$$

$$\text{where} \quad P = \frac{K \, D}{h} \tag{4}$$

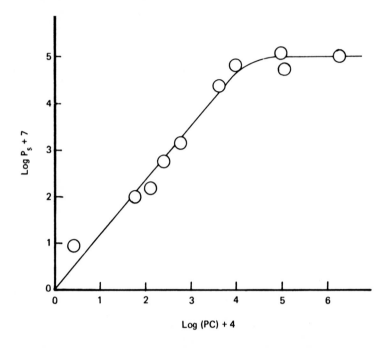

FIGURE 3.   Dependency of transdermal permeability P_s on partition coefficient (P.C.) of drugs in mineral oil-water system. Key: a, ouabain; b, atropine; c, digitoxin; d, scopolamine; e, diethylcarbamazine; f, chlorpheniramine; g, ephedrine; h, nitroglycerin; i, estradiol; j, fentamyl.[87]

P and D are the permeability coefficient and the diffusion coefficient, respectively, and ΔC is the concentration difference between the drug concentrations in the two chambers.

For the trilaminate membrane illustrated by Figure 2, the overall coefficient may be expressed as follows:

$$P = \cfrac{1}{\cfrac{1}{P_{SC}} + \cfrac{1}{P_E} + \cfrac{1}{P_D}} \qquad (5)$$

where P_{SC}, P_E, and P_D are the permeability coefficients of the stratum corneum, the epidermis, and the dermis, respectively. As the permeability coefficients are the reciprocals of the diffusional resistances, the denominator in Equation 5 may be written as:

$$R = R_{SC} + R_E + R_D \qquad (6)$$

where R is the overall diffusional resistance of the skin to the permeation of a compound and R_{SC}, R_E, and R_D are the diffusional resistances of the stratum corneum, the epidermis, and the dermis, respectively. Examples of the effect of partition coefficient on skin permeability[87] are given in Figure 3. A variety of drug substances are shown to give a good correlation between their skin permeabilities and their mineral oil-water partition coefficients when aqueous media are the solvents in the donor and receiver chambers. The skin permeability increases when the partition coefficient increases until a partition coefficient of about one is reached; thereafter the skin permeability appears to plateau with further increase of the partition coefficient.

The stratum corneum, being much more lipoidal than the epidermis and dermis, is apparently the rate-limiting step for the permeation of polar substances which have low partition coefficients. In other words, $P_{SC} \ll P_E$ or P_D for polar substances. Therefore, Equation 5 becomes:

$$P \cong P_{SC} = \frac{K_{SC} D_{SC}}{h_{SC}} \qquad (7)$$

A direct proportion between the permeability coefficient and the partition coefficient is therefore maintained. On the other hand, for the highly lipophillic substances, $P_{SC} \gg P_E$ or P_D. Equation 5 then becomes:

$$P = \frac{1}{\dfrac{1}{P_E} + \dfrac{1}{P_D}} \qquad (8)$$

and the epidermis and the dermis may become rate limiting in the case of highly lipophilic substances. The epidermis and the dermis are believed to be essentially aqueous, and therefore P_E and P_D may be insensitive to partition coefficient changes. When the stratum corneum is removed, Equation 8 prevails for both the polar and nonpolar substances, as is shown in Figure 4.[88] The transition from Equation 7 and Equation 8 is illustrated in Figure 4 (partial removal of the stratum corneum).

The partition coefficient of a compound can be increased conveniently and economically by increasing the alkyl chain length of a homologous series. A linearity is often observed between the logarithm and the alkyl chain length:

$$\log K_n = \log K_o + \pi_n \qquad (9)$$

For most organic solvents, the values of π vary only slightly from solvent to solvent in which the partition coefficients are measured. As a rule of thumb, $\pi = 0.5$ is generally satisfactory. The values of π for several organic solvents are listed in Table 9.[89]

The changes in partition coefficient between a parent compound and its lowest member derivative upon prodrug formation are shown in Table 10. It is interesting to note that the lowest member derivative does not always improve the partition coefficient over the parent compound. Conversion of an aromatic hydroxyl group to an acetate ester gives no increase in the partition coefficient whereas conversion of an aliphatic carboxyl group to the methyl ester gives rise to an increase in the partition coefficient equivalent to adding two methylene groups. Conversely, conversion of an aromatic acid to the corresponding amide results in a decrease in the partition coefficient equivalent to removing 2.5 methylene groups. Homologation by methylene group addition can be conveniently used to increase the partition coefficient of a compound. More complete tables of the influence of structure modification on the partition coefficient are available in the literature.[90]

B. Biological Considerations

Skin is known to be a metabolically active membrane.[91] The viable epidermis, which contains most of the catabolic enzymes that might render a drug inactive by metabolism, is metabolically more active than dermis.[92,93] For a transdermally delivered drug, the drug molecule must overcome the metabolic barrier of the skin to become systemically available. It was reported that more than 95% of the testosterone absorbed was metabolized as it permeated through the skin.[94] Table 11 lists various types of bioconversion which may occur in the skin and the skin enzymes involved.

Prodrugs, on the contrary, may overcome the metabolic barrier to achieve the systemic bioavailability or make use of the skin bioconversion to reduce the systemic toxicity for

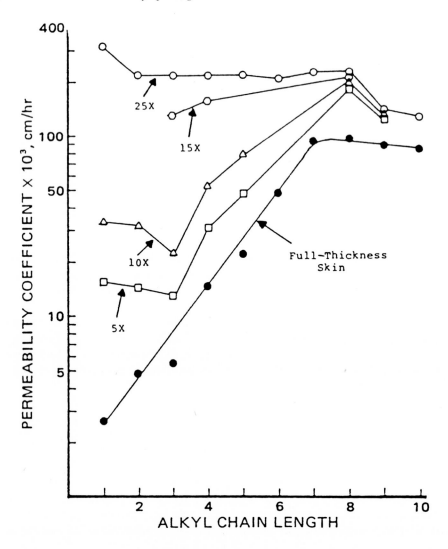

FIGURE 4.   Semilog plot of permeability coefficients for stripped hairless mouse membranes and normal hairless mouse skin as a function of alkyl chain length. All data were obtained at 37°. The skin was stripped 5, 10, 15 and 25 times.[88]

topical therapies. A fine example of the latter is fluocortin butyl ester (FCB).[91] In contrast to other corticosteroid esters, FCB is bioconverted to systemically inactive metabolites. This bioconversion leads to a safer use of FCB in the topical corticoid therapy for infants, pregnant women, and the elderly because of the reduced systemic toxicity.

IV. EXPERIMENTAL EVALUATION OF TRANSDERMALLY DELIVERED PRODRUGS

The purpose of this section is to describe a methodology which combines in vitro diffusion cell experiments with freshly excised animal skin and theoretical techniques for describing and quantifying the transport and metabolism of prodrugs in this membrane. A quantitative model has been developed which treats the skin as a three-layer membrane (stratum corneum, epidermis, and dermis). Diffusivity values are assigned to the prodrug, drug, and the metabolite for each layer. Enzyme parameters are also assigned for each layer. The model with a single set of these parameter values has been shown to be in very good agreement with

Table 9[a]
VALUES OF π_{CH_2} FOR
SOME COMMON
SOLVENTS

Solvent	π_{CH_2}
Ether	0.573
Ether	0.612
Octanol	0.500
Chloroform	0.609
Olive oil	0.525
Castor oil	0.545

[a] Taken from Reference 89.

experimental data on the transport and metabolism of the ester prodrugs of ara-A (ara-A-acetate, ara-A-valerate, and ara-A-octanoate) in excised hairless mouse skin. Finally, the model parameters (the diffusivities and the enzyme parameters) have been validated by independent experiments.

This approach should prove to be valuable in evaluating the performance of and, more importantly, in the rational design of prodrugs in dermal drug delivery problems as drug fluxes, species concentration profiles, and where in the skin, the relevant biochemical events occur can easily be predicted or mapped out from the results of the analysis.

A. The Model and Equations for the Transport/Metabolism of the 5'-Monoesters of ara-A in the Hairless Mouse Skin

Figure 5 schematically illustrates the hairless mouse skin which is comprised of the stratum corneum (h $\simeq$ 10 to 20 μ), the epidermis (h $\simeq$ 4 to 50 μ), and the dermis (h $\simeq$ 250 μ). In the skin, we have the following scheme for the enzymatic reactions:

$$A \text{ (prodrug)} \xrightarrow{\text{esterase}} B \text{ (drug)} \xrightarrow{\text{deaminase}} C \text{ (metabolite)}$$

In the quasisteady-state, we may write the following equations which describe the (one-dimensional) simultaneous enzymatic reactions and diffusion:

$$D_{A,i} \frac{d^2 [A]}{d X^2} - \frac{V_{m,i} [A]}{K_m + [A]} = 0 \tag{10}$$

$$D_{B,i} \frac{d^2 [B]}{d X^2} + \frac{V_{m,i} [A]}{K_m + [A]} - \frac{V'_{m,i} [A]}{\left(1 + \frac{[A]}{K_I}\right) K'_m + [B]} = 0 \tag{11}$$

$$D_{C,i} \frac{d^2 [C]}{d X^2} + \frac{V'_{m,i} [B]}{\left(1 + \frac{[A]}{K_I}\right) K'_m + [B]} = 0 \tag{12}$$

The D's are the diffusivities. The subscripts A, B, and C refer to the three species and i refers to the ith component, or stratum of the membrane. The coordinate X is the perpendicular depth in the membrane. V_m and K_m are the Michaelis-Menten kinetics parameters for the esterase and V'_m and K'_m are those for the deaminase. K_I is the deaminase inhibition constant for the prodrug.[95] For the general case, the D's, K_m's, V_m's, and the K_I's may all

Table 10[a]
LIPOPHILICITY CHANGE UPON PRODRUG FORMATION OF COMMON FUNCITONAL GROUPS ON THE *n*-OCTANOL/WATER SCALE

	Drug	Example derivative	$\Delta \pi$	ca. CH_2 group equiv
			Lipophilicity change	
Esters	Aliphatic R–OH	$\text{R–O–}\overset{\displaystyle O}{\overset{\|}{C}}\text{–CH}_3$	+ 0.82	+ 1.5
	Aromatic R–OH	$\text{R–O–}\overset{\displaystyle O}{\overset{\|}{C}}\text{–CH}_3$	+ 0.03	0
	Aliphatic $\text{R–}\overset{\displaystyle O}{\overset{\|}{C}}\text{–OH}$	$\text{R–}\overset{\displaystyle O}{\overset{\|}{C}}\text{–O–CH}_3$	+ 0.99	+ 2
	Aromatic $\text{R–}\overset{\displaystyle O}{\overset{\|}{C}}\text{–OH}$	$\text{R–}\overset{\displaystyle O}{\overset{\|}{C}}\text{–O–CH}_3$	+ 0.27	+ 0.5
Amides	Aliphatic $\text{R–}\overset{\displaystyle O}{\overset{\|}{C}}\text{–OH}$	$\text{R–}\overset{\displaystyle O}{\overset{\|}{C}}\text{–NH}_2$	− 0.45	− 1
	Aromatic $\text{R–}\overset{\displaystyle O}{\overset{\|}{C}}\text{–OH}$	$\text{R–}\overset{\displaystyle O}{\overset{\|}{C}}\text{–NH}_2$	− 1.21	− 2.5
	Aromatic R–NH_2	$\text{R–NH–}\overset{\displaystyle O}{\overset{\|}{C}}\text{–CH}_3$	+ 0.36	+ 0.75
	Aliphatic R–NH_2	$\text{R–NH–}\overset{\displaystyle O}{\overset{\|}{C}}\text{–CH}_3$	+ 0.52	+ 1
Ethers	Aliphatic R–OH	R–O–CH_3	+ 0.69	+ 1.25
	Aromatic R–O–H	R–O–CH_3	+ 0.65	+ 1.25

[a] Taken from reference 23.

be functions of X. It is, however, shown that, although the parameter values may be different for the different components of a membrane, e.g., epidermis, dermis, and stratum corneum, they may be assumed to be constant within a particular membrane component.

At low concentration of the prodrug, Equations 10 to 12 reduce to:

$$D_{A,i} \frac{d^2 [A]}{d X^2} - k_i [A] \tag{13}$$

$$D_{B,i} \frac{d^2 [B]}{d X^2} + k_i [A] - k_i' [B] = 0 \tag{14}$$

Table 11[a]
BIOCONVERSIONS IN HUMAN SKIN

Reaction	Phase I — Reactions	Substrate
	Enzymes involved	
Oxidation		
Aliphatic C—atoms	Mixed functions oxidase	7,12-Dimethylbenz(a)anthracene (DMBA)
Alicyclic C—atoms	Mixed function oxidase	Dehydroepiandrosterone (DHA) →7αOH-DHA, 7β OH-DHA
Aromatic rings	Hydroxylases	3,4-Benzopyrene (BP) → phenol → quinone → dihydrodiol
Alcohols	Hydroxysteroiddehydrogenases	Cortisol → cortisone testosterone → Δ⁴-androsteneβ-3,17-dione 17β-estradiol → estrone
Deamination	MAO	Norepinephrine
Dealkylation	Deethylase	7—Ethoxycoumarin
Reduction	Demethylase	Aminopyrine
Carbonyl groups	Ketoreductase	Cortisol → Reichstein's E, epi-E
		Progesterone → (Allo)pregnanediol
		Estrone → 17β-estradiol 5α-DHT, 5α-androstane-3α,17β-diol
		5α-androstane-3,17-dione → androsterone, epiandrosterone
–C=C–Double bonds	5α-Reductase	Testosterone → 5α-DHT
		Progesterone → 5α-DHP
Hydrolysis		
Ester bonds	Esterases	Diflucortolone-21-valerate Betamethasone-21-valerate Betamethasone-17-valerate Fluocortin-butylester
Epoxides	Epoxidehydratase (EH)	Styrene oxide
	Phase II — Reaction	
Glucuronide formation	UDPG-transferase	Benz(a)pyrene o-aminophenol
Sulfate formation	Sulfo-transferase	DHA Δ⁵-Androstene-3β,17β-diol
Methylation	COMT	Norephinephrine
Glutathione conjugation	Glutathion-S-transferase	Styrene glycol

ᵃ   Taken from Reference 91.

$$D_{C,i} \frac{d^2 [C]}{d X^2} + k_i' [B] = 0 \qquad (15)$$

Much of the model development studies and model validation studies were conducted using tracer levels of substrates and Equations 13 to 15.

B. Analysis of the Model with Experimental Data

Diffusion cell experiments[96,97] using full thickness hairless mouse skin, stripped skin (Scotch® tape removal of stratum corneum) and dermis skin yielded permeability coefficients.

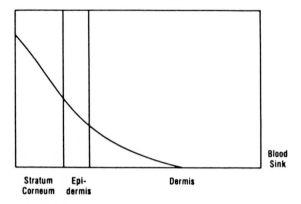

FIGURE 5.   The multilayer model for simultaneous diffusion and metabolism of drug in the skin.

Table 12
PERMEABILITY COEFFICIENTS OF ara-A, A-ara-A, V-ara-A,
AND O-ara-A THROUGH WHOLE SKIN

Mouse Number	Permeability coefficient × 10⁸ (cm/sec)				
	ara-A	A-ara-A	V-ara-A	O-ara-A	Ester/ara-A
0621797	0.74	0.90	—	—	1.21
0621798	0.93	1.18	—	—	1.26
0714802	0.81	0.97	—	—	1.20
0714803	0.65	0.84	—	—	1.30
0621797	0.74	—	1.39	—	1.87
0621798	0.93	—	1.92	—	2.06
0714802	0.81	—	1.47	—	1.81
0714803	0.65	—	1.34	—	2.07
0621797	0.74	—	—	3.22	4.33
0621798	0.93	—	—	3.37	3.61
0714802	0.81	—	—	3.42	4.22
0714803	0.65	—	—	3.01	4.65

Table 12 shows the permeability coefficients of ara-A and its three monoesters for full thickness skin. Moderate increases in permeability coefficients are seen with increases in lipophilicity of the prodrug. Stripped skin permeabilities are listed in Table 13. Permeability coefficients are around 100 times larger when the stratum corneum is removed. The moderate influence of lipohilicity upon the permeability coefficient is still present when the stratum corneum is removed. The diffusivity (D) values may be calculated from the relation $D = P \cdot h$, where P is the permeability coefficient and h is the thickness for the membrane component in question.

1. Validation Studies

Model validation studies were conducted for tracer levels of all three ester prodrugs. Equations 13 to 15 were solved numerically using experimental D-values and thickness for each of the membrane components. Data were obtained in a two-chamber cell for the simultaneous transport and bioconversion as described previously.[96,97] Tables 14 and 15 give the back diffusion fluxes and forward fluxes of prodrug and drug for ara-A-acetate, ara-A-valerate, and ara-A-octanoate. Tables 16, 17, and 18 show the best fit of the calculated data to the experimental fluxes for ara-A-acetate, ara-A-valerate, and ara-A-octanoate, respectively. The fitting involved deducing the best set of k_i and k_i' values.

Table 13
PERMEABILITY COEFFICIENTS OF ara-A, A-ara-A, V-ara-A,
AND O-ara-A IN STRIPPED SKIN

Mouse number	Permeability coefficient $\times$ 10^6 (cm/sec)				
	ara-A	A-ara-A	V-ara-A	O-ara-A	Ester/ara-A
0405802	1.25	1.90	—	—	1.52
0417802	1.19	0.82	—	—	1.53
0405802	1.25	—	3.78	—	3.02
0417802	1.19	—	3.67	—	3.08
0405802	1.25	—	—	8.11	6.49
0417802	1.19	—	—	7.98	6.71

Table 14
OBSERVED FLUXES IN GO-THROUGH EXPERIMENT WITH A-ara-A
$\rightarrow$ V-ara-A $\rightarrow$ O-ara-A USING STRIPPED SKIN FROM A 12-WEEK-OLD
MOUSE

Order of run[a]	Direction[b]	Prodrug	Flux/initial donor conc $\times$ 10^6 (cm/sec)			
			Donor		Receiver	
			Prodrug	ara-A	Prodrug	ara-A
1	Epidermis $\rightarrow$ dermis	A-ara-A	—	1.12	1.37	0.77
2	Epidermis $\rightarrow$ dermis	V-ara-A	—	3.64	1.24	2.26
3	Epidermis $\rightarrow$ dermis	O-ara-A	—	16.70	1.55	6.86

Note: #0417804A, Skin was soaked and rinsed for 2 hr before the first run.

[a]   Indicates the 1st, 2nd, or 3rd run with the given skin preparation.
[b]   Indicates the permeation direction, i.e., the donor side to the receiver side.

Table 15
OBSERVED FLUXES IN GO-THROUGH EXPERIMENT WITH A-ara-A
$\rightarrow$ V-ara-A $\rightarrow$ O-ara-A USING STRIPPED SKIN FROM A 12-WEEK-OLD
MOUSE

Order of run[a]	Direction[b]	Prodrug	Flux/initial donor conc $\times$ 10^6 (cm/sec)			
			Donor		Receiver	
			Prodrug	ara-A	Prodrug	ara-A
1	Dermis $\rightarrow$ epidermis	A-ara-A	—	7.05	1.17	0.69
2	Dermis $\rightarrow$ epidermis	V-ara-A	—	22.30	1.16	2.15
3	Dermis $\rightarrow$ epidermis	O-ara-A	—	59.00	1.14	5.03

Note: #0417804B, Skin was soaked and rinsed for 2 hr before the first run.

[a]   Indicates the 1st, 2nd, or 3rd run with the given skin preparation.
[b]   Indicates the permeation direction, i.e., the donor side to the receiver side.

Table 16
LEAST SQUARES FITTING OF THE CALCULATED FLUXES TO THE EXPERIMENTAL DATA FOR THE DETERMINATION OF THE ESTERASE RATE CONSTANTS (BASED ON THE DATA IN TABLES 14 AND 15)

	Flux/initial donor conc × 10^6 (cm/sec)							
	Epidermis → dermis[a] (1st run)				Dermis → epidermis[a] (2nd run)			
	Donor		Receiver		Donor		Receiver	
	V-ara-A	ara-A	V-ara-A	ara-A	V-ara-A	ara-A	V-ara-A	ara-A
Expt. data	—	3.64	1.24	2.26	—	22.3	1.16	2.15
Best fit[b]	—	3.96	1.18	2.63	—	23.7	1.18	2.21

[a]   Indicates the permeation direction, i.e., the donor side to the receiver side.
[b]   Iteration parameters:

$k_{epi} = 1.21 \times 10^{-2}$/sec $k_{dermis} = 1.63 \times 10^{-3}$/sec
$D_{PDepi} = 4.90 \times 10^{-9}$ cm²/sec $D_{Depi} = 3.10 \times 10^{-9}$ cm²/sec
$h_{epi} = 1.0 \times 10^{-3}$ cm $h_{dermis} = 2.5 \times 10^{-2}$ cm
$D_{dermis} = 5.3 \times 10^{-7}$ cm²/sec

Table 17
LEAST SQUARES FITTING OF THE CALCULATED FLUXES TO THE EXPERIMENTAL DATA FOR THE DETERMINATION OF THE ESTERASE RATE CONSTANTS (BASED ON DATA IN TABLES 14 AND 15)

	Flux/initial donor conc × 10^6 (cm/sec)							
	Epidermis → dermis[a] (1st run)				Dermis → epidermis[a] (2nd run)			
	Donor		Receiver		Donor		Receiver	
	A-ara-A	ara-A	A-ara-A	ara-A	A-ara-A	ara-A	A-ara-A	ara-A
Expt. data	—	1.12	1.37	0.77	—	7.05	1.17	0.69
Best fit[b]	—	0.98	1.39	0.67	—	6.95	1.27	0.68

[a]   Indicates the permeation direction, i.e., the donor side to the receiver side
[b]   Iteration parameters:

$k_{epi} = 2.52 \times 10^{-3}$/sec $k_{dermis} = 2.96 \times 10^{-4}$/sec
$D_{PDepi} = 3.22 \times 10^{-9}$ cm²/sec $D_{Depi} = 2.61 \times 10^{-9}$ cm²/sec
$h_{epi} = 1.0 \times 10^{-3}$ cm $h_{dermis} = 2.5 \times 10^{-2}$ cm
$D_{dermis} = 5.3 \times 10^{-7}$ cm²/sec

Direct experimental values for k_i and k_i' in the epidermis and dermis were obtained by the use of trypsin to separate the dermis from the epidermis. Tissue homogenization of the separated components yielded k_i and k_i' in the epidermis and dermis for ara-A and its three monoesters (Table 19). Examining Table 20, it can be seen that for all three monoesters, the rate constants in the epidermis are 8 to 10 times higher than in the dermis. This is in agreement with the results previously obtained[96] for ara-A-valerate.

The good agreement between the directly obtained experimental homogenate values and the model deduced values in the epidermis is seen in Table 20. Table 21 shows the good agreement between experimental and model-deduced enzyme constants in the dermis.

After completing the model validation studies for tracer levels (Equations 13 to 15), the

Table 18
LEAST SQUARES FITTING OF THE CALCULATED FLUXES TO THE EXPERIMENTAL DATA FOR THE DETERMINATION OF THE ESTERASE RATE CONSTANTS (BASED ON THE DATA IN TABLES 14 AND 15)

	Flux/initial donor conc $\times$ 10^6 (cm/sec)							
	Epidermis $\to$ dermis[a] (1st run)				Dermis $\to$ epidermis[a] (2nd run)			
	Donor		Receiver		Donor		Receiver	
	O-ara-A	ara-A	O-ara-A	ara-A	O-ara-A	ara-A	O-ara-A	ara-A
Expt. data	—	16.7	1.55	6.86	—	59.0	1.14	5.03
Best fit[b]	—	14.8	1.43	8.02	—	49.8	1.16	5.18

[a] Indicates the permeation direction, i.e., the donor side to the receiver side.
[b] Iteration parameters:

$k_{epi} = 5.03 \times 10^{-2}$/sec
$D_{PDepi} = 1.61 \times 10^{-8}$ cm²/sec
$h_{epi} = 1.0 \times 10^{-3}$ cm
$D_{dermis} = 5.3 \times 10^{-7}$ cm²/sec

$k_{dermis} = 4.87 \times 10^{-3}$/sec
$D_{Depi} = 3.79 \times 10^{-9}$ cm²/sec
$h_{dermis} = 2.5 \times 10^{-2}$ cm

Table 19
COMPARISON OF ESTERASE AND ADENOSINE DEAMINASE ACTIVITIES IN THE EPIDERMIS AND DERMIS OF THE HAIRLESS MOUSE SKIN

		Specific enzymatic activity $\times$ 10^3 (1/sec/g of tissue)			
		Deaminase	Esterase		
Mouse number	Fraction of membrane	ara-A	A-ara-A	V-ara-A	O-ara-A
1027806	Epidermis	9.62	2.33	13.30	43.10
	Dermis	1.54	0.25	1.41	5.20
1201802	Epidermis	7.75	2.60	11.20	47.00
	Dermis	1.20	0.32	1.51	5.90
1201804	Epidermis	7.62	2.71	15.50	56.60
	Dermis	1.41	0.31	1.77	4.15

validity of the model when prodrug levels were near saturated solution concentrations (Equations 10 to 12) was established. The results of saturated go-through experiments are presented in Tables 22, 23, and 24 for ara-A-acetate, ara-A-valerate and ara-A-octanoate, respectively. In these experiments, the first and third runs were always tracer levels with the second run having saturated or near-saturated drug concentrations. The above sequence of runs allowed for direct comparison of the effect, if any, of using saturated drug concentrations.

Model validation studies with high concentrations of the prodrugs entailed determining the K_m, K'_m, and K_I values for all three prodrugs with the homogenates. $V_{m,i}$ and $V'_{m,i}$ values were then calculated from $(V_{m,i}/K_m) = k_i$ and $(V'_{m,i}/K'_m) = k'_i$. These parameters values were then used in Equations 10 to 12 and fluxes were numerically calculated for the two-chamber diffusion cell experiments. It should be noted that all variables except diffusivities

Table 20

COMPARISON OF EPIDERMIS ESTERASE RATE CONSTANTS OBTAINED FROM MODEL FITTING AND THOSE OBTAINED FROM TRYPSIN TREATMENT

Prodrug	$K_{trypsin} \times 10^3$ (1/sec/g of tissue)	$K_{model} \times 10^3$ (1/sec/g of tissue)	$\dfrac{K_{trypsin}}{K_{e\ acetate}}$	$\dfrac{K_{model}}{K_{e\ acetate}}$
A-ara-A	2.3—2.7	2.5—3.5	1	1
V-ara-A	11.2—15.5	10.6—13.5	4.3—5.7	3.8—4.3
O-ara-A	43.1—56.6	46.3—56.8	17.1—20.8	16.1—18.6
ara-A	7.6—9.6[a]	6.5—9.3[a]	—	—

[a] Deminase constants.

Table 21

COMPARISON OF DERMIS ESTERASE RATE CONSTANT OBTAINED FROM MODEL FITTING TO THOSE OBTAINED FROM TRYPSIN TREATMENT

Prodrug	$K_{trypsin} \times 10^4$ (1/sec/g of tissue)	$K_{model} \times 10^4$ (1/sec/g of tissue)	$\dfrac{K_{trypsin}}{K_{d\ acetate}}$	$\dfrac{K_{model}}{K_{d\ acetate}}$
A-ara-A	2.5—3.1	2.8—3.1	1	1
V-ara-A	14.1—17.7	11.3—15.2	4.5—7.0	4.8—5.4
O-ara-A	41.5—59.0	41.9—45.7	13.2—23.4	13.3—16.4
ara-A	1.2—1.5[a]	1.4—1.6[a]	—	—

[a] Deaminase constants.

Table 22

GO-THROUGH EXPERIMENT WITH SATURATED A-ara-A SOLUTION (#0418811)

Order of runs[a]	Flux/initial donor conc $\times 10^6$ (cm/sec)					
	Donor			Receiver		
	A-ara-A	ara-A	ara-H	A-ara-A	ara-A	ara-H
1st[b]	—	0.82	0.24	1.72	0.19	0.57
2nd[c]	—	0.59	0.08	1.55	0.37	0.23
3rd[b]	—	0.82	0.25	1.77	0.19	0.58

[a] All runs were conducted with epidermis facing the donor chamber.
[b] Only trace amounts of ^{3}H-A-ara-A were used in these two runs.
[c] Saturated A-ara-A solution ($2.69 \times 10^{-2}M$) spiked with trace amount of ^{3}H-A-ara-A was used in this run.

were determined independently, the diffusivities being obtained directly from permeability experiments. Tables 25, 26, and 27 show the reasonably good agreement obtained between the calculated and experimentally determined fluxes for ara-A-acetate, ara-A-valerate, and ara-A-octanoate.

It can be concluded that both esterase and deaminase enzymes are quantitatively accounted for by the model with the diffusivities obtained in the permeability experiments.

Table 23
GO-THROUGH EXPERIMENTS WITH SATURATED
V-ara-A SOLUTION (#0418812)

Order of runs[a]	Flux/initial donor conc × 10^6 (cm/sec)					
	Donor			Receiver		
	V-ara-A	ara-A	ara-H	V-ara-A	ara-A	ara-H
1st[b]	—	2.28	0.87	1.13	0.54	1.62
2nd[c]	—	0.84	0.21	1.19	0.59	0.83
3rd[b]	—	2.31	0.87	1.12	0.55	1.66

[a] All runs were conducted with epidermis facing the donor chamber.
[b] Only trace amounts of ^{3}H-V-ara-A were used in these two runs.
[c] Saturated V-ara-A solution (2.39×10^{-2} M) spiked with trace amount of ^{3}H-V-ara-A was used in this run.

Table 24
GO-THROUGH EXPERIMENT WITH SATURATED O-ara-A
SOLUTION (#0418813)

Order of runs[a]	Flux/initial donor conc × 10^6 (cm/sec)					
	Donor			Receiver		
	O-ara-A	ara-A	ara-H	O-ara-A	ara-A	ara-H
1st[b]	—	6.68	10.20	1.08	1.15	4.65
2nd[c]	—	10.20	5.88	1.18	1.77	3.37
3rd[b]	—	6.70	10.20	1.13	1.17	4.71

[a] All runs were conducted with epidermis facing the donor chamber.
[b] Only trace amounts of ^{3}H-O-ara-A were used in these two runs.
[c] Saturated O-ara-A solution (5.85×10^{-4}M) spiked with trace amount of ^{3}H-O-ara-A was used in this run.

2. Concentration-Distance Profiles

Having validated the model and having obtained the appropriate transport and metabolism parameters for ara-A, ara-A-acetate, ara-A-valerate, and ara-A-octanoate, concentration-distance profiles can now be obtained from Equations 10 to 12 or 13 to 15. These calculated species concentrations are expected to be the actual aqueous steady-state concentrations and therefore may be directly considered in the drug efficacy predictions.

The plots in Figures 6 and 7 represent, the epidermal concentration-distance profiles for ara-A valerate in whole skin and stripped skin, respectively, when saturated solutions are topically applied. Similar plots for ara-A-acetate and ara-A-octanoate have also been obtained.[97] The fifth and eight rows in Table 28 give the steady-state drug and metabolite concentrations for ara-A and its three monoesters in whole skin and stripped skin when saturated solutions are topically applied. It can be seen (upperhalf of Table 28) that for whole skin, the incorporation of Michaelis-Menten kinetics and/or the prodrug-inhibition consideration have only small effects. With saturated prodrug or drug concentrations, the low permeabilities of ara-A and its three monoesters through the stratum corneum preclude the buildup of high-enough prodrug and drug concentration for saturation of esterase or deaminase to be important in the epidermis. It can be concluded that for whole skin, the enzymatic reactions can be well approximated with first-order kinetics even when saturated

Table 25

FITTING OF EXPERIMENTAL FLUXES FROM GO-THROUGH EXPERIMENTS USING THE PHYSICAL MODEL (#0418811)

	Flux/initial donor conc $\times$ 10^6 (cm/sec)							
	Donor				**Receiver**			
	A-ara-A	ara-A + ara-H	ara-A	ara-H	A-ara-A	ara-A + ara-H	ara-A	ara-H
Expt data	—	0.67	0.59	0.08	1.55	0.60	0.37	0.23
Calc data[a]	—	0.71	0.62	0.09	1.54	0.63	0.39	0.24

[a]   Parameters used in the calculations:
$D_{epi} = 1.1 \times 10^{-9}$ cm²/sec
$V_{m,epi}$ (esterase) $= 3.5 \times 10^{-5}$ mol/sec
$V_{m,dermis}$ (esterase) $= 5.0 \times 10^{-6}$ mol/sec
$h_{epi} = 1.0 \times 10^{-3}$ cm
K_m (esterase) $= 3.3 \times 10^{-2} M$
$k_1 = 2.3 \times 10^{-4} M$
$D_{dermis} = 5.0 \times 10^{-7}$ cm²/sec
$V'_{m,epi}$ (deaminase) $= 1.0 \times 10^{-5}$ mol/sec
$V'_{m,dermis}$ (deaminase) $= 1.5 \times 10^{-6}$ mol/sec
$h_{dermis} = 2.5 \times 10^{-2}$ cm
K'_m (deaminase) $= 3.3 \times 10^{-4} M$

Table 26

FITTING OF EXPERIMENTAL FLUXES FROM GO-THROUGH EXPERIMENT USING THE PHYSICAL MODEL (#0418812)

	Flux/initial donor conc $\times$ 10^6 (cm/sec)							
	Donor				**Receiver**			
	V-ara-A	ara-A + ara-H	ara-A	ara-H	V-ara-A	ara-A + ara-H	ara-A	ara-H
Expt data	—	1.05	0.84	0.21	1.19	1.42	0.59	0.83
Calc data[a]	—	1.02	0.83	0.19	1.16	1.37	0.57	0.79

[a]   Parameters used in the calculations:
$D_{epi} = 2.2 \times 10^{-9}$ cm²/sec
$V_{m,epi}$ (esterase) $= 2.9 \times 10^{-5}$ mol/sec
$V_{m,dermis}$ (esterase) $= 2.6 \times 10^{-6}$ mol/sec
$h_{epi} = 1.0 \times 10^{-3}$ cm
K_m (esterase) $= 1.08 \times 10^{-3} M$
$k_1 = 1.2 \times 10^{-5} M$
$D_{dermis} = 5.0 \times 10^{-7}$ cm²/sec
$V'_{m,epi}$ (deaminase) $= 1.0 \times 10^{-5}$ mol/sec
$V'_{m,dermis}$ (deaminase) $= 1.5 \times 10^{-6}$ mol/sec
$h_{dermis} = 2.5 \times 10^{-2}$ cm
K'_m (deaminase) $= 3.3 \times 10^{-4} M$

Table 27
FITTING OF EXPERIMENTAL FLUXES FROM GO-THROUGH EXPERIMENT USING THE PHYSICAL MODEL (#0418813)

Flux/initial donor conc $\times 10^6$ (cm/sec)

	Donor				Receiver			
	O-ara-A	ara-A + ara-H	ara-A	ara-H	O-ara-A	ara-A + ara-H	ara-A	ara-H
Expt data	—	16.0	10.2	5.88	1.18	5.14	1.77	3.37
Calc data[a]	—	16.1	10.1	6.03	1.15	5.05	1.72	3.33

[a] Parameters used in the calculations:

$D_{epi} = 5.8 \times 10^{-9}$ cm²/sec
$V_{m,epi}$ (esterase) $= 1.3 \times 10^{-5}$ mol/sec
$V_{m,dermis}$ (esterase) $= 1.0 \times 10^{-6}$ mol/sec
$h_{epi} = 1.0 \times 10^{-3}$ cm
K_m (esterase) $= 1.51 \times 10^{-4}M$
$k_I = 8.8 \times 10^{-7}M$
$D_{dermis} = 5.0 \times 10^{-7}$ cm²/sec
$V'_{m,epi}$ (deaminase) $= 1.0 \times 10^{-5}$ mol/sec
$V'_{m,dermis}$ (deaminase) $= 1.5 \times 10^{-6}$ mol/sec
$h_{dermis} = 2.5 \times 10^{-2}$ cm
K'_m (deaminase) $= 3.3 \times 10^{-4}M$

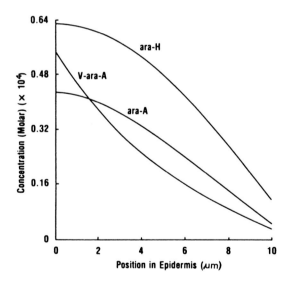

FIGURE 6.   Concentration-distance profile for ara-A-valerate in the epidermis of whole skin based on the model. The following parameters were used to generate the plot (values are listed in order of stratum corneum, epidermis, and dermis for each parameter).
   Diffusivity of ara-A-valerate: 6.8×10^{-11}, 3.9×10^{-9}, and 5.0×10^{-7} cm²/sec
   Diffusivity of ara-A and ara-H: 6.8×10^{-11}, 2.2×10^{-9}, and 5.0×10^{-7} cm²/sec
   Thickness: 40, 20, and 250 μm
   k_e: 0, 1.18×10^{-2} and 1.12×10^{-3} sec^{-1}
   k_d: 0, 7.4×10^{-3} and 1.5×10^{-3} sec^{-1}
   $K_{m,e}$: 1.1×10^{-3} M; $K_{m,d}$: 3.3×10^{-4} M; k_I: 1.2×10^{-5} M

70

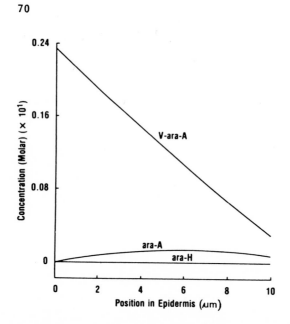

FIGURE 7.   Concentration-distance profile for ara-A-valerate in the epidermis of stripped skin based on the model. The following parameters were used to generate the plot (values are listed in order of epidermis and dermis for each parameter):

Diffusivity of ara-A-valerate: 3.9×10^{-9} and 5.0×10^{-7} cm²/sec

Diffusivity of ara-A and ara-H: 2.2×10^{-9} and 5.0×10^{-7} cm²/sec

k_e: 1.2×10^{-2} and 1.1×10^{-3} sec^{-1}

k_d: 7.4×10^{-3} and 1.5×10^{-3} sec^{-1}

$K_{m,e}$: 1.1×10^{-3} M; $K_{m,d}$: 3.3×10^{-4} M; k_l: 1.2×10^{-5} M

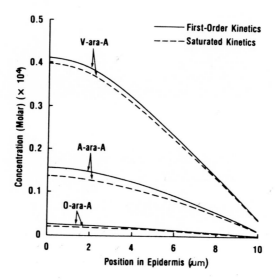

FIGURE 8.   Concentration-distance profiles of ara-A from topically applied saturated solutions of ara-A-acetate, ara-A-valerate, and ara-A-octanoate in hairless mouse full thickness skin. Parameter values taken from model validation studies.

Table 28
CALCULATED STEADY-STATE DRUG AND METABOLITE CONCENTRATION IN WHOLE SKIN AND STRIPPED SKIN

		Steady-state concentrations					
		Drug			Metabolite		
Compound	Interface	First-order kinetics	Enzyme saturation only	Enzyme saturation and prodrug inhibition	First-order kinetics	Enzyme saturation only	Enzyme saturation and prodrug inhibition
Whole skin							
Ara-A	Sc/epi[a]	2.0×10^{-6}	2.0×10^{-6}	—	2.7×10^{-6}	2.7×10^{-6}	—
	Epi/dermis[b]	6.5×10^{-8}	6.5×10^{-8}	—	4.0×10^{-7}	4.0×10^{-7}	—
Ara-A-acetate	Sc/epi	1.4×10^{-5}	1.4×10^{-5}	1.6×10^{-5}	2.3×10^{-5}	2.3×10^{-5}	2.1×10^{-5}
	Epi/dermis	1.7×10^{-6}	1.7×10^{-6}	1.9×10^{-6}	4.4×10^{-6}	4.4×10^{-6}	4.2×10^{-6}
Ara-A-valerate	Sc/epi	3.9×10^{-5}	4.2×10^{-5}	3.9×10^{-5}	6.4×10^{-5}	6.1×10^{-5}	6.3×10^{-5}
	Epi/dermis	4.2×10^{-6}	4.4×10^{-6}	4.4×10^{-6}	1.2×10^{-5}	1.2×10^{-5}	1.2×10^{-5}
Ara-A-octanoate	Sc/epi	1.9×10^{-6}	$1.9 \ 10^{-6}$	2.0×10^{-6}	3.1×10^{-6}	3.0×10^{-6}	3.1×10^{-6}
	Epi/dermis	2.9×10^{-7}	$2.9 \ 10^{-7}$	1.9×10^{-7}	5.6×10^{-7}	5.5×10^{-7}	5.7×10^{-7}
Stripped skin							
Ara-A	Sc/epi	1.3×10^{-3}	1.3×10^{-3}	—	3.3×10^{-9}	1.2×10^{-9}	—
	Epi/dermis	4.0×10^{-5}	6.1×10^{-5}	—	6.1×10^{-5}	6.3×10^{-5}	—
Ara-A-acetate	Sc/epi	1.9×10^{-8}	1.5×10^{-8}	1.6×10^{-8}	5.1×10^{-9}	1.3×10^{-9}	1.6×10^{-10}
	Epi/dermis	3.8×10^{-4}	4.7×10^{-4}	6.0×10^{-4}	4.0×10^{-4}	1.8×10^{-4}	4.5×10^{-5}
Ara-A-valerate	Sc/epi	7.0×10^{-8}	8.7×10^{-9}	9.9×10^{-9}	1.7×10^{-8}	1.2×10^{-9}	1.1×10^{-11}
	Epi/dermis	1.2×10^{-3}	6.4×10^{-4}	8.3×10^{-4}	1.3×10^{-3}	2.0×10^{-4}	3.7×10^{-6}
Ara-A-octanoate	Sc/epi	6.4×10^{-9}	2.3×10^{-9}	2.8×10^{-9}	1.5×10^{-8}	5.4×10^{-10}	8.4×10^{-12}
	Epi/dermis	9.7×10^{-5}	9.3×10^{-5}	1.6×10^{-4}	1.1×10^{-4}	6.5×10^{-5}	2.6×10^{-6}

[a] Stratum corneum-epidermis boundary.
[b] Epidermis-dermis boundary.

drug solutions are applied on the surface of the membrane. The bottom half of Table 28 similarly examines the cases for stripped skin. It can be seen that the effects of enzyme saturation and prodrug inhibition of deaminase are roughly of the same order of magnitude (about $\pm$ a factor of 2) for all three prodrugs. By examining Table 28, the reader may evaluate more critically the relative importances of esterase saturation, deaminase saturation, and the prodrug inhibition of deaminase for each of the prodrugs. Figures 8 and 9 present plots of the steady-state ara-A concentrations based on these calculations for the saturated solution cases.

The example presented here is that for the monoester prodrugs of ara-A in the hairless mouse skin. The quantitative self-consistency between the model and the experimental results demonstrates that this approach should be considered in dermal prodrug delivery research when there is simultaneous transport and metabolism of the prodrug.

V. TOXICOLOGICAL AND REGULATORY CONSIDERATIONS FOR TRANSDERMALLY DELIVERED PRODRUGS

Prodrugs are generally regarded as new drugs by regulatory agencies of a majority of countries.[98] Regulatory requirements for local and systemic toxicity testings in animals, skin irritation and sensitization testings in animals and humans, pharmacokinetic studies of the absorbed species, and clinical trials will be expected. However, in the case that the absorbed species is predominantly the parent drug which has been safely marketed for years, the systemic toxicity testings and pharmacokinetic studies of the absorbed species may be waived on a case-by-case basis.

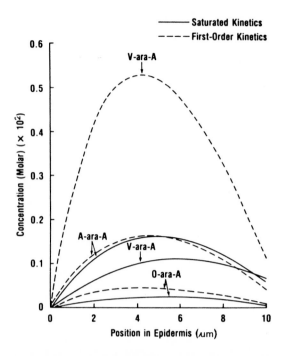

FIGURE 9.   Concentration-distance profiles of ara-A from topically applied saturated solutions of ara-A-acetate, ara-A-valerate, and ara-A-octanoate in hairless mouse stripped skin. Parameter values taken from validation studies.

REFERENCES

1. **Chien, Y.,** Logics of transdermal controlled drug administration, *Drug Dev. Ind. Pharm.,* 9, 497, 1983.
2. **Chien, Y., Keshary, P. R., Huang, Y. C., Sarpotdar, P. O.,** Comparative controlled skin permeation of nitroglycerin from marketed transdermal delivery systems, *J. Pharm. Sci.,* 72, 968, 1983.
3. **Chandrasekaran, S. K. and Shaw, J. E.,** Design of transdermal therapeutic systems, in *Contemporary Topics in Polymer Science,* Vol. 2, Pearce, E. M. and Schaefgen, J. R., Eds., Plenum Press, New York, 1977, 291.
4. **Chandrasekaran, S. K. and Shaw, J. E.,** Controlled transdermal delivery, in *Controlled Release of Bioactive Materials,* Baker, R., Ed., Academic Press, New York, 1980, 99.
5. **Shaw, J. E.,** Transdermal therapeutic systems, in *1st Int. Symp. Dermal and Transdermal Absorption,* Brandau, R. and Lippold, B. H., Eds., Wissenschaftliche Verlagsgesellschaft, Stuttgart, Germany, 1982, 171.
6. **Zaffaroni, A.,** Industrial development of transdermal therapeutic systems, in *1st Int. Symp. Dermal and Transdermal Absorption,* Brandau, R. and Lippold, B. H., Eds., Wissenschaftliche Verlagsgesellschaft, Stuttgart, Germany, 1982, 188.
7. **Zaffaroni, A.,** Therapeutic Implications of Controlled Drug Delivery, presented at the 6th Int. Congr. Pharmacology, Helsinki, Finland, 1975.
8. **Shaw, J.,** Development of transdermal therapeutic systems, *Drug Dev. Ind. Pharm.,* 9, 579, 1983.
9. **Chandrasekaran, S. K., Bayne, W., and Shaw, J. E.,** Pharmacokinetics of drug permeation through human skin, *J. Pharm. Sci.,* 67, 1370, 1978.
10. **Good, W. R.,** Transderm-Nitro: controlled delivery of nitroglycerin via the transdermal route, *Drug Dev. Ind. Pharm.,* 9, 647, 1983.
11. **Karim, A.,** Transdermal absorption: a unique opportunity for constant delivery of nitroglycerin, *Drug Dev. Ind. Pharm.,* 9, 671, 1983.
12. **Chien, Y. W., Rozek, L. F., and Lambert, H. J.,** Microsealed drug delivery systems. I. In vitro-in vivo correlation on subcutaneous release of desoxycorticosterone acetate and prolonged hypertensive animal model for cardiovascular studies, *J. Pharm. Sci.,* 67, 214, 1978.

13. **Chien, Y. W. and Lambert, H. J.,** U.S. Patent 3,946,106, 1976.
14. **Chien, Y. W. and Lambert, H. J.,** U.S. Patent 3,992,518, 1976.
15. **Chien, Y. W. and Lambert, H. J.,** U.S. Patent 4,053,580, 1977.
16. **Keith, A. D. and Snipes, W.,** Eur. Patent 0,013,606, 1980.
17. **Zierenberg, B.** (Boehringer Ingelheim), Ger. Offen. DE 3,204,551, 1983; *Chem. Abstr.,* 99, 181471s, 1983.
18. Nitto Electric Industrial Co. Ltd., Jpn. Kohai Tokyo Koho JP 58,128,324 [83,129,324], 1983; *Chem Abstr.,* 99, 181473u, 1983.
19. **Keith, A. and Snipes, W.,** (Key Pharmaceuticals, Inc.), Belg. BE 889,549, 1981; *Chem. Abstr.,* 96, 110174z, 1982.
20. Sekisui Chemical Co. Ltd., Jpn. Kokai Tokyo Koho JP 58,138,462 (83,138,462), 1983; *Chem. Abstr.,* 99, 200563s, 1983.
21. **Sinkula, A. A. and Yalkowsky, S. H.,** Rationale for design of biologically reversible drug derivatives: prodrugs, *J. Pharm. Sci.,* 64, 111, 1975.
22. **Stella, V. J.,** Prodrugs: An overview and definition, in *Prodrugs as Novel Drug Delivery Systems,* Higuchi, T. and Stella, V., Eds., ACS Symposium Series No. 14, American Chemical Society, Washington, D.C., 1975, 1.
23. **Ho, N. F. H., Park, J. Y., Morozowich, W., and Higuchi, W. I.,** Physical model approach to the design of drugs with improved intestinal absorption in *Design of Biopharmaceutical Properties through Prodrugs and Analogs,* Roche, E. B., Ed., American Pharmaceutical Association, Washington, D.C., 1977, 136.
24. **Sinkula, A. A.,** Methods to achieve sustained drug delivery, *The Chemical Approach in Sustained and Controlled Release Drug Delivery Systems,* Robinson, J. R., Ed., Marcel Dekker, New York, 1978, 411.
25. **Stella, V. J., Mikkelson, T. J., and Pipkin, D.,** Prodrugs: the control of drug delivery via bioreversible chemical modification, in *Drug Delivery Systems. Characteristics and Biomedical Applications,* Juliano, R. L., Ed., Oxford University Press, New York, 1980, 112.
26. **James, K. C., Nicholls, P. J. and Roberts, M.,** Biological half-lives of [4-^{14}C] testosterone and some of its esters after injection into the rat, *J. Pharm. Pharmacol.,* 21, 24, 1969.
27. **Sinkula, A.A.,** The chemical approach to achieve sustained drug delivery in *Optimization of Drug Delivery,* Alfred Benzon Symposium 17, Bundgaard, H., Hansen, A. B., and Kofod, H. Eds., Munksgaard, Copenhagen, Denmark, 1982, 199.
28. **Albert, A.,** Chemical aspects of selective toxicity, *Nature (London),* 182, 421, 1958.
29. **Albert, A.,** *Selective Toxicity,* 3rd ed., Wiley and Sons, New York, 1964, 57.
30. **Harper, N. J.,** Drug latentiation, *J. Med. Pharm. Chem.,* 1, 467, 1959.
31. **Harper, N. J.,** Drug latentiation, *Progr. Drug Res.,* 4, 221, 1962.
32. **Harper, N. J.,** in *Absorption and Distribution of Drugs,* Binns, T. B., Ed., Williams and Wilkins, Baltimore, 1964, 103.
33. **Ariens, E. J.,** Molecular pharmacology, a basis for drug design, *Progr. Drug Res.,* 10, 429, 1966.
34. **Ariens, E. J.,** Modulation of pharmacokinetics by molecular manipulation, in *Drug Design,* Vol. 2, Ariens, E. J., Ed., Academic Press, New York, 1971, 2.
35. **Morozowich, W., Cho, M. J., and Kezdy, F. J.,** Application of physical organic principles to prodrug design, in *Design of Biopharmaceutical Properties through Prodrugs and Analogs,* Roche, E. B., Ed., American Pharmaceutical Association, Washington, D.C., 1977, 344.
36. **Sinkula, A. A.,** Prodrug approach in drug design, *Ann. Rep. Med. Chem.,* 10, 306, 1975.
37. **Sinkula, A. A.,** Perspective on prodrugs and analogs in drug design, in *Design of Biopharmaceutical Properties through Prodrugs and Analogs,* Roche, E. B., Ed., American Pharmaceutical Association, Washington, D.C., 1977, 1.
38. **von Daehne, W., Godtfredsin, W. V., Roholt, K., and Tybring, L.,** Pivampicillin, a new orally active ampicillin ester, *Antimicrob. Agents Chemother.,* 6, 431, 1970.
39. **McClure, D. A.,** The effect of a prodrug of epinephrine (di-pivalyl epinephrine) in glaucoma-general pharmacology, toxicology and clinical experience, in *Prodrug as Novel Drug Delivery Systems,* Higuchi, T. and Stella, V. J., ACS Symposium Series No. 14, American Chemical Society, Washington, D.C., 1975, 224.
40. **Bodor, N., Shek, E., and Higuchi, T.,** Delivery across the blood-brain barrier of a quaternary pyridinium salt (2-PAM) in a prodrug form, *Science,* 190, 155, 1975.
41. **Bodor, N., Shek, E., and Higuchi, T.,** Improved delivery through biological membranes. I. Synthesis and properties of 1-methyl-1, 6-dihydropyridine-2-aldoxime: a prodrug of 2-PAM, *J. Med. Chem.* 19, 102, 1976.
42. **Miescher, K., Wettstein, A., and Schopp, E. T.,** The activation of the male sex hormones. II, *Biochem. J.,* 30, 1977, 1936.
43. **Edgerton, W. H., Maddox, V. H., and Controulis, J.,** The structure of chloramphenicol palmitate, *J. Am. Chem. Soc.,* 77, 27, 1955.

44. **Sinkula, A. A., Morozowich, W., and Rowe, E. L.,** Chemical modification of clindamycin: synthesis and evaluation of selected esters, *J. Pharm. Sci.,* 62, 1106, 1973.

45. **Misher, A., Adams, H. J., Fisher, J. J., and Jones, R. G.,** Pharmacology of the hexylcarbonate of salicylic acid, *J. Pharm. Sci.,* 57, 1128, 1968.

46. **Morozowich, W., Lamb, D. C., DeHaan, R. M., and Gray, J. E.,** Clindamycin-2-phosphate, an injectable derivative of clindamycin with improved muscle tolerance, Abstract, Am. Pharm. Assoc. Academy of Pharmaceutical Sciences, 1977, 63.

47. **Morozowich, W., Oesterling, T. O., Miller, W. L., Lawson, C. F., Weeks, J. R., Stehle, R. G., and Douglas, S. L.,** Prostaglandin prodrugs. I. Stabilization of dinoprostone (prostaglandin E_2) in solid state through formation of crystalline C_1-phenyl esters, *J. Pharm. Sci.,* 68, 833, 1979.

48. **Amidon, G. L., Pearlman, R. S., and Leesman, G. D.,** Design of prodrugs through consideration of enzyme-substrate specificities, in *Design of Biopharmaceutical Properties through Prodrug and Analogs,* Roche, E. B., Ed., American Pharmaceutical Association, Washington, D.C., 1977, 281.

49. **Krisch, K.,** Carboxylic esterhydrolases, in *The Enzymes,* Vol. V, 3rd ed., Boyer, P. D., Ed., Academic Press, New York, 1971, 43.

50. **Croft, D. N., Cuddigan, J. H. P., and Sweetland, C.,** Gastric bleeding and benorylate, a new aspirin, *Br. Med. J.* 3, 545, 1972.

51. **Loftsson, T. and Bodor, N.,** Improved delivery through biological membranes X: percutaneous absorption and metabolism of methylsulfinylmethyl 2-acetoxybenzoate and related aspirin prodrugs, *J. Pharm. Sci.,* 70, 756, 1981.

52. **Hussain, A., Yamasaki, M., and Truelove, J. E.,** Kinetics of hydrolysis of acylals of aspirin: hydrolysis of (1'-ethoxy) ethyl 2-acetoxybenzoate, *J. Pharm. Sci.,* 63, 627, 1974.

53. **Truelove, J. E., Hussain, A. A., and Kostenbauder, H. B.,** Synthesis of 1-0-(2'acetoxy) benzoyl-α-D-2-deoxygluco-pyranose, a novel aspirin prodrug, *J. Pharm. Sci.,* 69, 231, 1980.

54. **Hussain, A., Truelove, J. E., and Kostenbauder, H.,** Kinetics and mechanism of hydrolysis of 1-(2'-acetoxybenzoyl)-2-deoxy-α-D-glucopyranose, a novel aspirin prodrug, *J. Pharm. Sci.,* 68, 299, 1979.

55. **Morozowich, W., Oesterling, T. O., Miller, W. L., and Douglas, S. L.,** Prostaglandin prodrugs. II. New method for synthesizing prostaglandin prodrugs. II. New method for synthesizing C_1-aliphatic esters, *J. Pharm. Sci.,* 68, 836, 1979.

56. **Weeks, J. R., DuCharme, D. W., Magee, W. E., and Miller, W. L.,** The biological activity of the (15S)-15-methyl analogs of prostaglandins E_2 and $F_2\alpha$, *J. Pharmacol. Exp. Ther.,* 186, 67, 1973.

57. **Thorp, J. M. and Waring, W. S.,** Modification of metabolism and distribution of lipids by ethyl chlorophenoxyiso-butyrate, *Nature (London),* 194, 948, 1962.

58. **Chang, I. H., Pinson, R. J., and Malone, M. H.,** Displacement of L-thyroxine from its binding proteins in human, dog and rat plasma by α-(p-chlorophenoxy) isobutyric acid, *Biochem. Pharmacol.,* 16, 2053, 1967.

59. **Holysz, R. P. and Stavely, H. E.,** Carboxy derivatives of benzylpencillin, *J. Am. Chem. Soc.,* 72, 4760, 1950.

60. **Daehne, W. V., Frederiksen, E., Gundersen, E., Lund, F., Morch, P., Peterson, H. J., Roholt, K., Tybring, L., and Godtfredson, W. O.,** Acyloxymethyl esters of ampicillin, *J. Med. Chem.,* 13, 607, 1970.

61. **Bodin, N. O., Ekstrom, B., and Forsgren, Y.,** Bacampicillin: a new orally well absorbed derivative of ampicillin, *Antimicrob. Agents Chemother.,* 8, 518, 1975.

62. **Clayton, J. P., Cole, M., Elson, S. W., and Ferres, H.,** BRL8988 (Talampicillin), a well absorbed oral form of ampicillin, *Antimicrob. Agents Chemother.,* 5, 670, 1974.

63. **Hobbs, D. C.,** Metabolism of indamyl carbenicillin by dogs, rats, and humans, *Antimicrob. Agents Chemother.,* 2, 272, 1972.

64. American Home Products, 2-amido-cephalosporins, U.S. Patent 2,748,328, 1973.

65. **Sinkula, A. A.,** Application of the prodrug approach to antibiotics, in *Prodrugs as Novel Drug Delivery Systems,* Higuchi, T. and Stella, V., Eds., ACS Symposium Series No. 14, American Chemical Society, Washington, D.C., 1975, 116.

66. **Glazko, A. J., Carnes, H. E., Kazenko, A., Wolf, L. M., and Reutner, T. F.,** Succinic acid esters of chloramphenicol, *Antibiot. Annu.,* 793, 1957.

67. **Ross, S., Puig, J. R., and Zaremba, E. A.,** Chloramphenicol acid succinate (sodium salt). Some preliminary clinical and laboratory observations in infants and children, *Antibiot. Annu.,* 803, 1957.

68. **Sandman, B.,** The Chemistry of Chloramphenicol 3-Monosuccinate, Ph.D. thesis, University of Wisconsin, Madison, 1968.

69. **Sandman, B., Szulczewski, D., Windheuser, J., and Higuchi, T.,** Rearrangement of chloramphenicol 3-monosuccinate, *J. Pharm. Sci.,* 59, 427, 1970.

70. **Kauffman, R. E., Shoeman, D. W., and Wan, S. H.,** Absorption and excretion of clindamycin-2-phosphate in children after intramuscular injection, *Clin. Phramacol. Ther.,* 13, 704, 1972.

71. **Sinkula, A. A., Morozowich, W., Lewis, C., and MacKellar, F. A.,** Synthesis and bioactivity of lincomycin-7-monoesters, *J. Pharm. Sci.,* 58, 1389, 1969.
72. **Morozowich, W., Cho, M. J., and Kezdy, F. J.,** Application of physical organic principles to prodrug design, in *Design of Biopharmaceutical Properties through Prodrugs and Analogs,* Roche, E. B., Ed., American Pharmaceutical Association, Washington, D.C., 1977, 344.
73. **Morozowich, W., Lamb, D. J., Karnes, H. A., Mackeller, F. A., Lewis, C., Stern, K. F., and Rowe, E. L.,** Synthesis and bioactivity of lincomycin-2-phosphate, *J. Pharm. Sci.,* 58, 1485, 1969.
74. **Dittert, L. W., Caldwell, H. C., Ellison, T., Irwin, G. M., Rivard, D. E., and Swintosky, J. V.,** Carbonate ester prodrugs of salicylic acid. Synthesis, solubility characteristics, in vitro enzymatic hydrolysis rates, and blood levels of total salicylate following oral administration to dogs, *J. Pharm. Sci.,* 57, 828, 1968.
75. **Davidson, I. W. F., Rollins, F. O., DiCarlo, F. J., and Miller, H. S.,** The pharmacodynamics and biotransformation of pentaerythritol trinitrate in man, *Clin. Pharmacol. Ther.,* 12, 972, 1971.
76. **Needleman, P., Lang, S., and Johnson, E. M., Jr.,** *J. Pharmacol. Exp. Ther.,* 181, 489, 1972.
77. **Litchfield, M. H.,** *J. Pharm. Sci.,* 60, 1599, 1971.
78. **Repta, A. J. and Hack, J.,** Acetaminophen prodrugs: 2-(*p*-acetaminophenoxy) tetrahydropyran, *J. Pharm. Sci.,* 62, 1892, 1973.
79. **Hussain, A. and Rytting, J. H.,** Prodrug approach to enhancement of rate of dissolution of allopurinol, *J. Pharm. Sci.,* 63, 798, 1974.
80. **Ercoli, A., Gardi, R., and Bruni, G.,** Ether derivatives of steroid hormones, in *Research Progress in Organic, Biological, and Medicinal Chemistry,* Vol. 1, Gallo, U. and Santamaria, L., Eds., Societa Editoriale Farmaceutica, Milan, Italy, 1964, 155.
81. **Beckett, A. H., Taylor, D. C., and Gorrod, J. W.,** Triaklyl-silyl moieties as potential pharmacokinetics modifying groups for aminoalcohols, *J. Pharm. Pharmacol.,* 27, 588, 1975.
82. **Bondesson, G., Hedborn, C., Magnusson, O., and Stjernstrom, N. E.,** Potential hypolipidemic agents. XIII. Synthesis and plasma lowering properties of some acetals derived from pyridylemethanol or nicotinaldehye. *Acta Pharm. Suec.,* 13, 1, 1976.
83. **Fouts, J. R., Kamm, J. J., and Brodie, B. B.,** Enzymatic reduction of prontosil and other azo dyes, *J. Pharmacol. Exp. Ther.,* 120, 291, 1957.
84. **Bloedow, D. C. and Hayton, W. L.,** Saturable first pass metabolism of sulfisoxazole N-acetyl in rats, *J. Pharm. Sci.,* 65, 334, 1976.
85. **Verbiscar, A. J. and Abood, L. G.,** Carbonate ester latentiation of physiologically active amines, *J. Med. Chem.,* 13, 1176, 1970.
86. **Wechter, W. J., Gish, D. T., Greig, M. E., Grey, D. G., Moxley, T. E., Kuentzel, S. L., Gray, L. G., Gibbons, A. J., Griffin, R. C., and Neil, G. L.,** Nucleic acids 16, orally active derivatives of ara-cytidine, *J. Med. Chem.,* 19, 1013, 1976.
87. **Michaels, A. S., Chandrasekaran, S. K., and Shaw, J. E.,** Drug permeation through human skin. Theory and in vitro experimental measurement, *A.I.Ch.E.J.,* 21, 985, 1975.
88. **Flynn, G. L., Durrheim, H., and Higuchi, W. I.,** Permeation of hairless mouse skin. II. Membrane section techniques and influence on alkanol permeabilities, *J. Pharm. Sci.,* 70, 52, 1981.
89. **Yalkowsky, S. H. and Flynn, G. L.,** Transport of alkyl homologs across synthetic and biological membranes: a new model for chain length-activity relationships, *J. Pharm. Sci.,* 62, 210, 1973.
90. **Dunn, W. J.,** Structural effects of partitioning behavior of drugs, in *Design of Biopharmaceutical Properties through Prodrugs and Analogs,* Roche, E. B., Ed., American Pharmaceutical Association, Washington, D.C., 1977, 47.
91. **Tauber, U.,** Metabolism of drugs on and in the skin, in *Dermal and Transdermal Absorption,* Brandan, R. and Lippold, B. H., Eds., Wissenschaftliche Verlagogesellschaft, Stuttgart, 1982, 133.
92. **Laerum, O. D.,** Oxygen consumption of basal and differentiating cells from hairless mouse epidermis, *J. Invest. Dermatol.,* 52, 204, 1969.
93. **Bamshad, J.,** Catechol-o-methyl transferase in epidermis, dermis and whole skin, *J. Invest. Dermatol.,* 52, 351, 1969.
94. **Marzulli, F. N., Brown, D. W. C., and Maibach, H. I.,** Techniques for studying skin penetration, *Toxicol. Appl. Pharmacol.,* (Suppl. 3), 76, 1969.
95. **Lipper, R. A., Machovech, S. N., Drach, J. C., and Higuchi, W. I.,** *Mol. Pharmacol.,* 14, 366, 1978.
96. **Yu, C. D., Gordon, N. A., Fox, J. L., Higuchi, W. I., and Ho, N. F. H.,** *J. Pharm. Sci.,* 69, 775, 1980.
97. **Gordon, N. A.,** Ph.D. thesis, University of Michigan, Ann Arbor, 1981.
98. **Higuchi, T.,** Prodrug, molecular structure and percutaneous delivery, in *Design of Biopharmaceutical Properties through Prodrugs and Analogs,* Roche, E. B., Ed., American Pharmaceutical Association, Washington, D.C., 1977, 409.

Chapter 4

DRUG STRUCTURE VS. PENETRATION

Bernard Idson and Charanjit R. Behl

TABLE OF CONTENTS

I. INTRODUCTION

In this chapter, an attempt is made to present data and discuss relatively recent results of skin permeability of test compounds, particular drug compounds, classes of drug compounds, and drug categories.

Katz and Poulsen,[1] and Reiss,[2] have ably summarized the percutaneous absorption of drugs prior to 1971. The diversity of reporting experimental results rendered difficult systematic treatment and correlation of data between compounds and even in different investigations of the same molecule. The results obtained from various existing methods used for measuring the in vivo penetration for a given product are rarely comparable. This is due essentially to the diversity of methodologies used, animal species,[3,4] and anatomical site,[5,6] concentration of the permeants used,[7] various vehicles used,[3,8] and duration of the experiment.[3] Furthermore, experience has shown that it is very difficult to extrapolate to humans, the results obtained with animals.[9,10] While some investigators claim close correlation between in vitro and in vivo data,[11,12] others are less positive.[13] In addition, quantitative data are expressed in different ways, i.e., as permeability coefficients, Kp, diffusion coefficients D, activities, fluxes, percent diffusion, percent absorbed, pharmacological response, residual concentration on the skin surface, rate of absorption, etc. These diversities have lessened in recent studies and permeability coefficients are emerging as the most useful parameter for comparative purposes. If one assumes that an "average" Kp value is 1×10^{-4} cm/hr, the following chart can be a useful guide in classifying rate of penetration:

Fast	$> 1 \times 10^{-3}$
Intermediate	
Above average:	1×10^{-3} to 1×10^{-4}
Below average:	1×10^{-4} to 1×10^{-5}
Slow	$< 1 \times 10^{-5}$

A major obstacle that confronts gathering comparative data is the lack of definition of the vehicle, i.e., a solvent, nature of a "fatty vehicle", or not listing the components of the preparation used in the skin penetration experiments. This chapter details considerations of this type. Suffice it to say that if a compound is applied topically in a vehicle, the rate of its absorption is considerably influenced by that of the vehicle, by the degree of its partitioning between the vehicle and the stratum corneum, and by its concentration in the vehicle. If the degree of partitioning is very small, the compound is absorbed along with the vehicle. If the partitioning is considerable, percutaneous absorption may be independent of that of the vehicle.[14-16] A highly topically potent analog, appropriately formulated, has the greatest potential for clinical success. A marginally topically potent analog, even when well compounded, may produce suboptimal clinical results. The relationships between chemical structure and potency as measured by some pharmacological or microbiological tests, on the one hand, and chemical structure and potency as related to topical clinical performance on the other, must be defined for each therapeutic class of compounds.[15]

The pharmacological effects of a particular compound can sometimes be used to investigate percutaneous absorption. Topical application of microgram quantities of steroids incorporated in a cream or an ointment base produces local vasoconstriction which is visible as blanching. The degree and extent of blanching by topical corticosteroids were suggested as indicators of percutaneous absorption and as means of comparing absorption and efficacy in tests for new steroids.[17,18] Further experience indicated that this method of testing was neither accurate nor reproducible; the degree of blanching was subject to "observer error" and was found to vary in the same individual at different times of day even though the same anatomical site was used. The surrounding vascular skin color and degree of pigmentation were found to interfere considerably with the interpretation of results. Dissolving the steroid in ethyl alcohol did not appreciably improve the reproducibility of the vasoconstriction.[19] Despite these limitations, this method gave a reasonably close approximation between vasoconstrictor ability and clinical efficacy.[20-22] The production of an area of anesthesia by a topically applied substance could be used as a means of detecting percutaneous absorption, but it is even more subject to error than the vasoconstriction test.[23]

Other pharmacological parameters have been found useful in determining percutaneous absorption and are still used occasionally in order to relate pharmacological action with rates of absorption measured by other tests, e.g., changes in serum cholinesterase have been used to compare the toxicity of parathion and paraoxon after dermal application.[24-26] Antibiotic assays using microbiological techniques are sensitive and accurate. Vickers[27] compared the percutaneous absorption of sodium fusidate and fusidic acid using these techniques with the results of absorption obtained by standard ^{14}C-labeling techniques. Both by in vivo and in vitro methods, the results were found to be very close confirming the reliability of the radioisotope techniques.[28]

As a result of the diversity of methods and expressions of data, the authors usually duplicate the data of other investigators and attempt to discuss them. Preference has been given to the measurements of flux, permeability, diffusion, or the percent of dose absorbed in contrast to pharmacological end points.

II. COMPOUNDS AND PERMEATION

A. Test Compounds: Alkanols and Alkanoic Acids

The use of some test permeants such as water, alkanols, alkanoic acids, etc. can be very useful in carrying out the mechanistic studies which can be explained on theoretical considerations. This can be particularly helpful in studying structure-permeability relationships. Higuchi[29] and Barry[14] have been particularly interested in the influence of drug structure on steps in the overall process of absorption-release of molecules from the solid state to the vehicle, e.g., for a suspension or ointment, and the clearance of penetrant from the viable epidermis below the barrier layer of the stratum corneum. They concluded that classical thermodynamics does not allow comparison of the relative maximal fluxes of a series of congeneric drugs. There is no method in classical thermodynamics in which, for example, n molecules of hydrocortisone can equal m molecules of betamethasone. However, for the purpose of drug design it would be useful to designate an infinitely dilute solution of an

Table 1
**APPROXIMATE THERMODYNAMIC ACTIVITIES OF
PURE COMPOUNDS FOR CORRELATION WITH
MAXIMAL PERCUTANEOUS DELIVERY**[29]

Compound	Activity of pure state[a] (mol/ℓ)	Compound	Activity of pure state[a] (mol/ℓ)
Methanol	0.1	Phenol	0.67
Ethanol	0.135	4-Iodophenol	1.56×10^{-2}
1-Butanol	0.20	4-Nitrophenol	3.6×10^{-4}
1-Hexanol	0.41	2,4,6-Triiodophenol	5×10^{-3}
Acetanilide	9×10^{-3}	Phthalic anhydride	5×10^{-4}
Benzene	11.2	Methyl testosterone	1.23×10^{-3}
Chloroform	12.4	Norethindrone	7.1×10^{-5}
Carbazole	1.5×10^{-3}	Norethindrone acetate	2.75×10^{-3}
Ethyl ether	9.55	Hydrocortisone	$<2 \times 10^{-6}$
Picric acid	3×10^{-4}	Hydrocortisone acetate	$<2 \times 10^{-6}$

[a]   Estimated values at 25°C with infinitely dilute solution in hexane, heptane,
or octane having activity coefficient of unity (1 M concentration).

alkane solvent as a reference state.[30] The approach may be used to predict structure-activity relationships for systems essentially at equilibrium or quasi-equilibrium such as steady-state skin permeation.[31]

Table 1 lists a variety of substances, together with their approximate thermodynamic activities in the pure state. Provided that all other factors are equal, theory predicts that the maximal expected rate of percutaneous delivery should correlate with the values of the activities given. On this basis, we would expect, for example, that chloroform and benzene would be delivered about a hundred times faster than the polar alcohols, methanol, and ethanol. Steroidal molecules, e.g., methyl testosterone or norethindrone and its acetate, should be delivered much more slowly than simple nonelectrolytes, and topical steroids such as hydrocortisone and hydrocortisone acetate should have low rates.

For most lipophilic drugs in water, activity coefficients are much greater than one. Table 2 lists the estimated activity coefficients of some common substances in dilute aqueous solution. One way of appreciating the usefulness of this data is to realize that, for example, for a long-chain alcohol such as 1-octanol, a 0.01 M solution in water has the same thermodynamic driving tendency for octanol as its 1 M solution in an alkane solvent such as isooctane. Similarly, for methanol a theoretical 200 M solution in water would be needed to provide the same driving tendency as the unit molar solution in isooctane. This is a thermodynamic way for quantifying the concept that at the same concentration of a drug, polar materials are released to the skin better from nonpolar solvents than from polar solvents; for nonpolar materials the reverse is true. For the extreme case listed in the table (octane), a 8.3×10^{-7} M solution in water is equivalent to the 1 M isooctane solution. Higuchi[29] concludes that clearance from the carrier as the rate-determining process probably does not become significant for drugs until their activity coefficient in water becomes greater than about 10^3 to 10^5.

Water, *n*-alkanols, and *n*-alkanoic acids are good test permeants because they are small, simple, metabolically stable molecules. While the molecular size and shape remain relatively constant, the alkanols experience almost a 100-fold increase in octanol/water partition coefficients in going from methanol to octanol. This provides an excellent source of chemicals to examine the influence of permeant lipophilicity on the percutaneous absorption with other factors remaining mostly invariant.

Table 2
ESTIMATED ACTIVITY COEFFICIENTS OF
ORGANIC COMPOUNDS IN WATER AT 25°C FOR
CORRELATION WITH CLEARANCE FROM THE
STRATUM CORNEUM BARRIER[29]

Compound	Activity coefficient[a]	Compound	Activity coefficient[a]
Alcohols		Phenol	0.70
Methanol	5.0×10^{-3}	Amines	
Ethanol	1.0×10^{-2}	Butylamine	0.76
1-Propanol	4.3×10^{-2}	Pentylamine	3.1
2-Propanol	2.7×10^{-2}	Hexylamine	13
1-Butanol	0.24	Octylamine	2.3×10^{2}
2-Butanol	0.11	Decylamine	4.1×10^{3}
2-Methyl 1-propanol	0.17	Alkanes	
2-Methyl 2-propanol	0.09	Pentane	1.2×10^{4}
1-Pentanol	0.98	Hexane	6.2×10^{4}
1-Hexanol	4.4	Heptane	2.5×10^{5}
1-Octanol	96	Octane	1.2×10^{6}
1-Decanol	210		

a   Based on activity coefficients in infinitely dilute solution in isooctane to be unity with concentrations in mol/ℓ.

Scheuplein and co-workers have extensively studied the permeability behaviors of water and *n*-alkanols through the human skin.[32-41] Table 3 contains data on the permeability coefficients, solubilities, partition coefficients, and the diffusion coefficients of alkanols. There is roughly a 150-fold increase in permeability from methanol to octanol. The classical diffusion theory would, however, predict a slight decrease in the actual mobility of the molecules on the basis of the fourfold increase in the molecular volume. The observed increase in permeability with an increase in the permeant molecular weight (Figure 1) emphasizes the overwhelming influence of the solubility term or the partition coefficient term.[32]

More recently, the permeability of *n*-alkanols and water has been studied using various animals' skins.[43-50] Data on the intact hydrated and un-hydrated hairless mouse skin,[45] stripped skins of hairless mice,[50] fuzzy rat skin,[46] and the *in situ* permeabilities of the hairless mouse[48] and fuzzy rat[47] skins are all shown in Table 4. Both in vitro as well as the *in situ* data show increased skin permeability with increase in the alkyl chain length of the permeants; an observation consistent with the human skin in vitro permeability discussed earlier.[38] Data from Table 4 were plotted semilogarithmically as permeability vs. alkyl chain length (Figure 2). All these plots demonstrate a sigmoidal shape showing three regions[51] (Figure 3): (1) an aqueous pore type pathway which may originate in the appendages or microchannels in the stratum corneum (Region I of Figure 3), (2) partitioning through the lipoidal components of the stratum corneum (Region II), and (3) diffusion through the aqueous strata, viable epidermis, and dermis (Region III). The data show that the profiles of the in vitro data for the hairless mouse and the fuzzy rat skins are comparable with the human skin data. The *in situ* data, however, shows the presence of only Regions I and II. The absence of Region III in the *in situ* data has mechanistic significance and may mean that the role of the aqueous strata in case of the *in situ* permeation is not important in controlling the rate of skin transport. This information is extremely important for the design of new drug molecules as well as for the development of topical formulations.

Recently, data on porcine skin permeability to alkanoic acids have been reported.[52,53] The

Table 3
ALCOHOL PERMEABILITY DATA FOR EPIDERMIS[38]

Molecule	kp (cm/hr)	$\triangle C_s$ (mol/ℓ)	J_s, µmol (cm²/hr)	K_m	D, cm² (sec × 10⁹)	Ref.
Aqueous solutions						
H_2O	0.5	0.1	0.05	0.88	0.57	157, 164
Methanol	0.5	0.1	0.05	0.6	0.62	
Ethanol	0.8	0.1	0.08	0.9	0.66	
Propanol	1.4	0.1	0.14	1.3	0.88	
Butanol	2.5	0.1	0.25	2.5	0.74	27, 34
Pentanol	6.0	0.1	0.60	5.0	0.88	
Hexanol	13.0	0.055	0.71	10.0	0.96	
Heptanol	32.0	0.015	0.48	30.0	0.79	
Octanol	52.0	0.0035	0.18	50.0	0.77	
Nonanol	60.0	0.0014	0.08			
Pure liquids						
H_2O	0.2	55.5	11.0	0.88	0.17	14, 26
Methanol	10.4	24.9	259.0	0.6	6.41	
Ethanol	0.72	17.1	12.3	0.9	0.30	
Propanol	0.12	13.3	1.6	0.6	0.07	
Butanol	0.06	10.9	0.65	0.25	0.09	34
Pentanol	0.051	9.2	0.47	0.11	0.17	
Hexanol	0.052	8.2	0.43	0.067	0.29	
Heptanol	0.025	7.1	0.18	0.063	0.15	
Octanol	0.010	6.3	0.06	0.028	0.13	
Nonanol	0.003	5.8	0.02			

Note: In both cases the receptor volumes were pure H_2O:alcohol (aq.) → water; alcohol (liq.) → water. Symbols: kp = permeability coefficient, $\triangle C_s$ = saturation solubility, J_s = flux, k_m = membrane vehicle partition coefficient, D = diffusion coefficient.

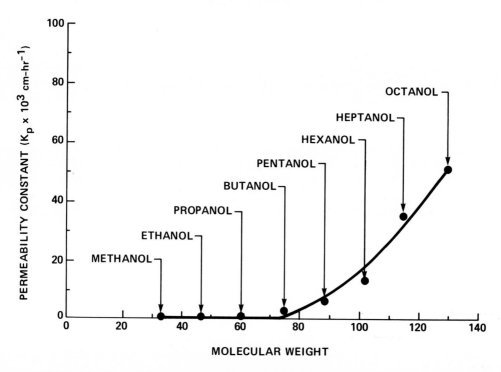

FIGURE 1.   Permeability constants of various primary alcohols when penetrating from saline.[32]

Table 4
PERMEABILITIES OF Δ-ALKANOLS THROUGH VARIOUS ANIMAL SKINS

Permeability coefficients $\times$ 10^3 (cm/hr)

| | In vitro | | | | *In situ* | |
| | Hairless mouse | | | Fuzzy rat | Hairless mouse | Fuzzy rat |
Permeant	Unhydrated	Hydrated	Stripped			
Reference	45	45	49	46	48	47
Water	1.3 ± 0.2	1.3 ± 0.2	420.0 ± 18.9	—	11.2 ± 2.4	—
Methanol	2.0 ± 0.4	2.0 ± 0.4	264.9 ± 20.7	1.9	27.8 ± 10.5	—
Ethanol	2.1 ± 0.1	2.1 ± 0.1	311.4 ± 22.0	2.2	30.9 ± 10.5	3.9 ± 1.1
Butanol	5.4 ± 1.1	9.7 ± 2.4	169.1 ± 22.0	8.4	39.9 ± 11.0	8.4 ± 2.1
Hexanol	19.4 ± 7.8	37.9 ± 11.7	302.5 ± 19.6	26.1	80.2 ± 8.1	31.6 ± 15.4
Octanol	78.2 ± 10.8	94.9 ± 15.0	207.4 ± 8.0	47.1	148.4 ± 14.6	159.0 ± 33.4
Decanol	—	—	—	—	400.3 ± 65.0	—

permeability coefficients were determined by using the alkanoic acids in their pure state as well as in nonaqueous solutions (Table 5). Semilogarithmic plots of these data (Figure 4) show almost linear exponential decline in the skin permeability. This is typical of permeability behavior from nonaqueous media. This can be compared with the permeability data obtained from the aqueous solutions of *n*-alkanoic acids[54] (Figure 5). The semilogarithmic profiles of these data are comparable to that of the alkanol data (Figure 2). Note that one set of data was obtained with pH 3.0 buffer on the donor side and pH 7 buffer on the receiver side, i.e., 3/7 system whereas the second set was obtained at 8/7 system. The first set of data represents consistently higher permeabilities which is consistent with the traditionally accepted pH-partition hypothesis according to which unionized species penetrate biological membranes much faster than the ionized species.

B. Linoleic Acid

Hoelgaard and Molgaard[55] determined the permeability of rat and human skins to free linoleic acid. The fatty acid is believed to aid in relieving the syndrome of essential fatty acid deficiency in persons suffering from fat malabsorption and in patients maintained on fat-free parenteral nutrition.

Table 6 shows that at the termination of the experiment (after 95 hr) the amount of linoleic acid within the human and the hairless rat skins was found to be 12 and 96 $\mu g/cm^2$, respectively. The data generated in this study showed that 8.6% dose diffuses into human skin and 55.6% dose diffuses into hairless rat skin in 95 hr. The flux obtained for human and rat skins was 0.036 and 0.098 $\mu g/cm^2/hr$, respectively. The rat skin was found to be about three times more permeable to linoleic acid than human skin, but either skin is relatively poorly permeable to the acid.

C. Alkyl Methyl Sulfoxides

A variety of organic solvents are known to influence the percutaneous passage of chemical agents but only few have been studied as intensively as dimethyl sulfoxide (DMSO).[23,28,56] The details of the use of DMSO is discussed in the chapter on percutaneous enhancers. Sekura and Scala[57] determined permeability coefficients for the penetration of an homologous series of alkyl methyl sulfoxides through guinea pig skin. These data are summarized in Table 7. The analogs were ranked in their permeabilities by comparing them against DMSO whose permeability was set equal to one. The data show that the alkyl chain length greatly influences the percutaneous penetration of the sulfoxides.

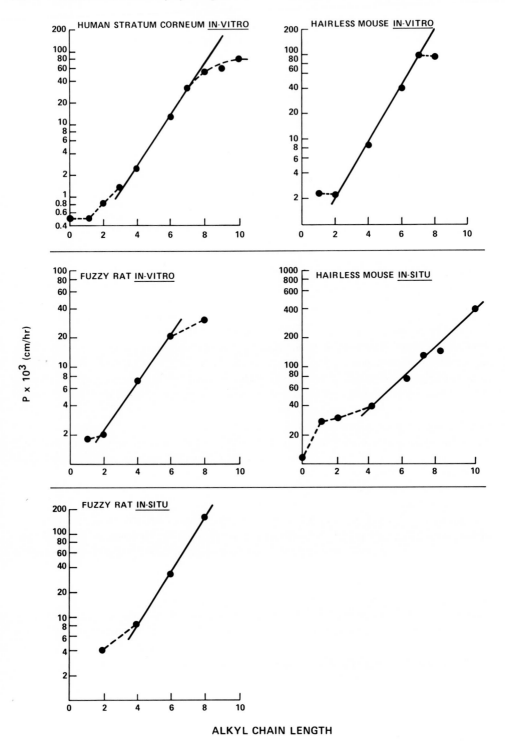

FIGURE 2.   Semilogarithmic plots of the skin permeability vs. the alkyl chain lengths.[38,45-48]

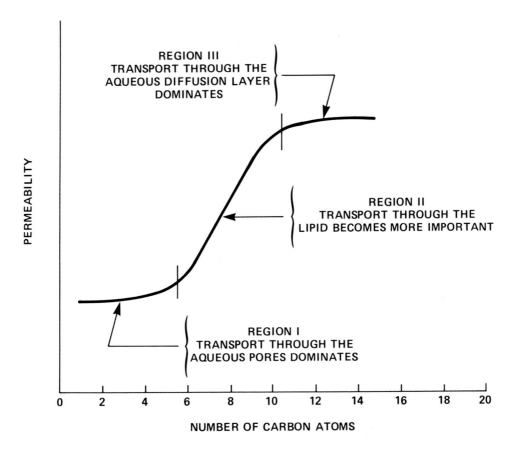

FIGURE 3.   Schematic representation of biological membrane permeability as a function of the alkyl chain length of the *n*-alkanols.[51]

Table 5
PERMEABILITIES OF *n*-
ALKANOIC ACIDS
THROUGH PORCINE SKIN[52,53]

Alkanoic acid	$P \times 10^3$ (cm/hr)	
	A	**B**
Acetic	8.4	351.6
Propionic	15.6	180.0
Butyric	15.0	60.0
Pentanoic	4.8	15.0
Hexanoic	1.2	4.8
Heptanoic	1.2	1.8
Octanoic	0.4	—

Note: (A) Permeation from pure alkanoic acids; (B) Permeation from dilute solutions of alkanoic acids in *n*-heptane.

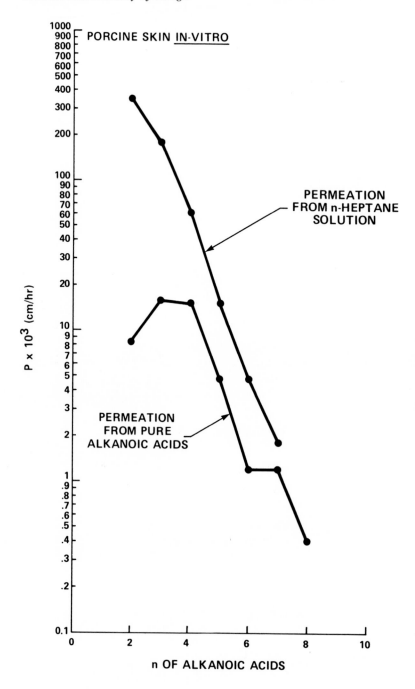

FIGURE 4.   Permeability of porcine skin to *n*-alkanoic acids.[52,53]

Except for the hexyl analog, which was less permeable than the decyl analog, the permeability decreases with an increase in the number of carbon atoms. Furthermore, the addition of a β-OH chain group to the C_{10} alkyl chain does not appreciably alter the skin permeability. This behavior is in contradiction to the generally accepted pattern of increased skin permeability with increasing the alkyl chain length, as was found with the *n*-alkanols described in Section II.A.

Sekura et al.[57] reported that the most reasonable explanation for the rapidly declining

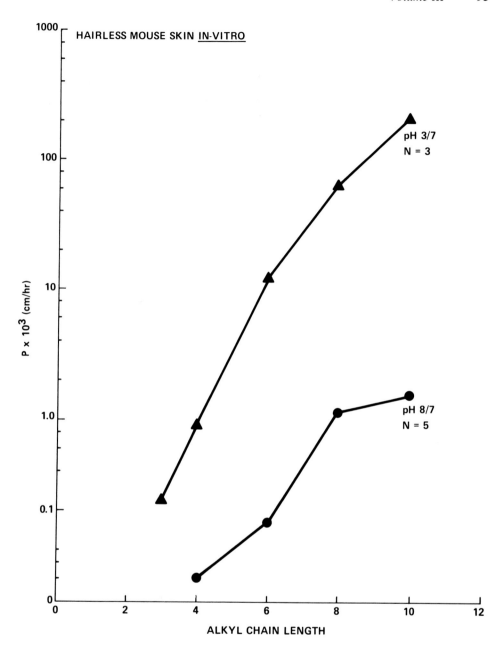

FIGURE 5.   Permeability of hairless mouse skin to *n*-alkanoic acids.[54]

penetration beyond $C_{10}MSO$ is that of decreasing water solubility and the presence of complex phases such as micelles and/or liquid crystals. The critical micelle concentrations of the long chain homologs in water are 10^{-3} M or less. Consistent with this is their observation that, in vitro, $C_{14}MSO$ penetrates better from an ethanolic solution in which it is more soluble than from water.

D. Benzoyl Peroxide

Nacht et al.[58] investigated the penetration and metabolic disposition of the antiacne agent, benzoyl peroxide. The study was performed in vitro with excised human skin and in vivo using the rhesus monkey.

Table 6

PERCUTANEOUS PERMEATION OF LINOLEIC ACID IN VITRO
(APPLIED DOSE OF 185 µg/cm²)[55]

	Flux µg/cm²/hr	In 95 hr		Total skin uptake	
		Total permeation µg/cm²	Amount in skin µg/cm²	µg/cm²	% dose
Human skin	0.036 ± 0.014	3.7 ± 1.5	12.1 ± 3.1	15.8	8.6
Hairless rat skin	0.098 ± 0.027	9.8 ± 2.3	96.0 ± 22.2	105.8	55.6

Table 7

PENETRATION OF SULFOXIDES THROUGH
EXCISED GUINEA PIG SKIN[57]

Sulfoxide	Permeability (cm/min) ($\times 10^{-4}$)	Relative permeability
DMSO	13	1
C_6-MSO	34	2.6
C_{10}-MSO	59	4.6
β-OH C_{10}-MSO	49	3.8
β-OH C_{12}-MSO	34	2.6
β-OH C_{14}-MSO	2.0	0.15
C_{14}MSO	1.5	0.11

Table 8

PERCUTANEOUS PENETRATION OF
BENZOYL PEROXIDE THROUGH EXCISED
HUMAN SKIN[58]

	µg[a]	%[b]	Chemical identity
Rinse (skin surface)	4350	95.5	Benzoyl peroxide
Soaks (skin layers)	120	2.6	Benzoyl peroxide and benzoic acid
Buffer (dermal side)	86	1.9	Benzoic acid
Total	4556	100.00	

[a]   Average of two diffusion cells.
[b]   Percent of the total amount recovered.

The results from the in vitro studies indicate that topically applied benzoyl peroxide penetrates the skin unchanged through the stratum corneum or through the follicular pathway (Table 8). The drug diffuses into the epidermis and the dermis, where it is converted, perhaps with the intervention of follicular bacteria, to benzoic acid. This metabolic conversion is apparently completed within the skin because the receptor buffer solution bathing the dermis contained only benzoic acid, the metabolic end product of benzoyl peroxide. Only 1.9% of the permeant penetrated through the skin and was recovered as benzoic acid in the receptor compartment of the diffusion cell. The skin retained 2.6% of the drug, about half of which was still intact. Thus, a total of 4.5% of the applied drug entered the skin and the remaining 95.5% remained on the surface of the skin. In the in vivo studies, following topical and intramuscular administration, 45 and 98% of the drug were recovered in the urine, respectively. Holzmann et al.[59] found that it was necessary to apply topically large amounts of

Table 9
COMPARISON IN DRUG RELEASE KINETICS AND SKIN PERMEATION PROFILES OF NITROGLYCERIN FROM PURE NITROGLYCERIN, TOPICAL 2% OINTMENT, AND CONTROLLED RELEASE TRANSDERMAL DELIVERY SYSTEMS[66]

	Loading dose (mg)	Surface area (cm²)	Flux or rate of release	Rate of skin permeation[a] (μg/cm²/hr)	% Loading dose delivered (24 hr)
Pure nitroglycerin	92.53	6.46	—	19.85 ± 3.4[b]	3.3 ± 0.6
2% ointment	5.3	2.8	187.3 ± 34.8[c] (μg/cm²/hr$^{1/2}$)	18.16 ± 3.4 (12 hr)[c] 14.44 ± 3.9 (12 hr)[c]	21.1 ± 2.64
Nitrodisc®	16.0	8.0	498.5 ± 27.8[b] (μg/cm²/hr$^{1/2}$	17.75 ± 2.8[c]	21.9 ± 3.9
Nitro-Dur®	51.0	10.0	841.6 ± 19.1[b] (μg/cm²/hr$^{1/2}$)	17.00 ± 2.8 (12 hr)[c] 10.34 ± 2.1 (12 hr)[c]	6.4 ± 1.2
Transderm-Nitro®	25.0	10.0	35.1 ± 2.9[b] (μg/cm²/hr)	14.10 ± 2.5[d]	13.9 ± 2.6
Deponit®	16.0	16.0	13.5 ± 0.9 (μg/cm²/hr)	7.30 ± 1.3[b]	19.4 ± 3.4

[a]   Mean ± standard deviation.
[b]   N = 4.
[c]   N = 8.
[d]   N = 12.

benzoyl peroxide (20 mg/cm²/day) to leg ulcers for 3 days before any benzoic acid was detected in the blood. It should be noted here that their assay method could detect only as low as 100 μg benzoic acid per milliliter of plasma.

E. Nitroglycerin

The outstanding example of transdermal delivery has been with the use of nitroglycerin (NTG) to avoid attacks of angina pectoris. Karim[60] has discussed the pharmacokinetics of transdermal absorption of NTG. He noted that NG is an ideal candidate for transdermal drug delivery. NTG is a potent, lipophilic, neutral compound with a low molecular weight. It undergoes extensive first-pass metabolism following oral administration.[61] NTG has a short elimination half-life of 2.8 min, a high apparent distribution volume of 3.3 ℓ/kg and a high plasma clearance of 0.72 ℓ/min/kg.[62]

Sublingually administered NTG has a rapid onset of action, but only for a short period of time, from 5 to 30 min.[63] This led to the use of topical formulations because it was long known that NTG is absorbed through the skin (as indicated by incidents in dynamite factories).[64] NTG, incorporated in an ointment base has a longer duration of action, 1 to 4 hours, but it has a delayed duration of action.[63]

Recently, Chien, Keshary, et al.[65,66] have studied the in vitro permeation of NTG from various systems, using the hairless mouse skin model. Their results indicate that despite wide variations in the systems, i.e., ranging from pure NTG to ointment to drug delivery patches marketed by four different manufacturers, the rate of skin permeation was invariant within a factor of two (Table 9). A maximal flux of 17.8 μg/cm²/hr was noted for Nitrodisc® and a minimal flux of 7.3 μg/cm²/hr was observed for Deponit®. Percent of loading dose penetrating in 24 hr varied from 3.3% for pure NTG to 21.9% for Nitrodisc®. The data in the hairless mouse skin model are generally comparable with the human skin data which indicate a flux in the range of 10 to 25 μg/cm²/hr.[67] These investigations stress the fact

Table 10
**PERMEATION STUDIES OF *N*-NITROSODIETHANOLAMINE IN
VARIOUS VEHICLES[68]**

Vehicle	Flux (ng/cm²/hr)	Permeability constant (cm/hr)	Membrane: vehicle partition coefficient
Water	7.1 ± 1.2	$5.5 \times 10^{-6}(6)^a$ $\pm 0.9 \times 10^{-6}$	1.8 ± 0.1(5)
Propylene glycol	4.7 ± 0.2	$3.2 \times 10^{-6}(5)$ $\pm 0.2 \times 10^{-6}$	1.0 ± 0.1(4)
Isopropyl myristate	292 ± 44	$1.1 \times 10^{-3}(9)$ $\pm 0.16 \times 10^{-3}$	228.2 ± 19.9(5)

[a]   Results are the mean ± SE of the number of determinations in parentheses.

that for designing a successful transdermal drug delivery system the drug needs to be highly lipophilic.

F. *N*-Nitrosodiethanolamine (NDELA)

NDELA is an impurity found in many cosmetic products and appears to be formed by a reaction between an amine such as diethanolamine or triethanolamine and a nitrosating agent. Since it has been found to be a carcinogen in animals, NDELA was examined for its ability to penetrate human skin.[68] The nitrosamine was applied to the skin in vehicles with different solubility properties (Table 10). The permeability constants for the vehicles, propylene glycol, and water (5.5×10^{-6} cm/hr), were small and similar in magnitude. In isopropyl myristate, the permeability constant increased approximately 250-fold to 1.1×10^{-3} cm/hr. The NDELA membrane/vehicle partition coefficients were determined using trypsin-treated stratum corneum as the membrane. These coefficients were 1.8 and 1.0, respectively, for water and propylene glycol and 230 for isopropyl myristate. The permeability of NDELA through the skin is apparently increased greatly when applied from sufficiently lipoidal formulations. This is primarily due to the favorable partitioning of the permeant from these formulations into the skin.

G. *p*-Hydroxybenzoates (Parabens)

Organic preservatives have affinities for both water and oil and are expected to penetrate into the skin easily.[69,70] Many studies have been concerned with the percutaneous absorption of preservatives, especially hexachlorophene.[71-75] However, there are only a few reports concerning the percutaneous absorption of the esters of *p*-hydroxybenzoic acid (parabens) despite their wide use as preservatives. Although it has been stated in the literature that parabens did not pass through a natural membrane 15 hr postapplication,[76] these substances must penetrate into the skin since they induce allergic reactions.[77,78]

Komatsu and Suzuki[79] studied the percutaneous absorption of aqueous butylparaben through excised guinea pig dorsal skin. The relative penetration of this compound decreases from system A-K (Table 11A and 11B). Although there was a small deviation in the diffusion constant in the 11 systems, no correlation was found between the system composition and the diffusion coefficients. Polysorbate 80 increased the solubilized concentration but decreased the penetration of the preservative. Polyethylene glycol 400 also reduced the amount of penetration. Propylene glycol was less effective than polyethylene glycol 400.

The partition coefficient varied significantly with the systems. Propylene glycol reduced the value significantly, but the effect was much less than that of polyethylene glycol 400. The effect of polysorbate 80 on the decrease of the partition coefficient was much more drastic. When polyethylene glycol 400 was co-existent with the surfactant, further reduction

Table 11A
THE EFFECT OF VEHICLE COMPOSITION ON PENETRATION OF BUTYLPARABEN[79]

System	Compound I, % (w/v)	Polysorbate 80, % (w/v)	Propylene glycol, % (v/v)	Polyethylene glycol 400, % (v/v)
A	0.015	—	—	—
B	0.02	—	10	—
C	0.02	—	—	10
D	0.02	—	20	—
E	0.02	—	—	20
F	0.1	1.0	—	—
G	0.1	1.0	10	—
H	0.1	1.0	—	10
I	0.1	2.0	—	—
J	0.1	2.0	10	—
K	0.1	2.0	—	10

Table 11B
VALUES OF DIFFUSION CONSTANT (D), PERMEABILITY CONSTANT (k_p), AND PARTITION COEFFICIENT (PC) OF THE STEADY-STATE PENETRATION AND PERCENTAGE PENETRATION OF THE TOTAL AMOUNT APPLIED

System	$D, \times 10^{-4}$ cm²/hr	$k_p, \times 10^{-4}$ cm/hr	PC	Penetration of total amount applied, %
A	3.43	70.82	2.77	23.70
B	4.53	53.70	1.59	20.22
C	4.26	16.76	0.53	5.70
D	3.38	26.88	1.07	9.54
E	3.04	7.52	0.33	1.95
F	3.28	9.36	0.38	3.64
G	3.34	12.04	0.48	3.54
H	3.46	7.08	0.27	2.17
I	3.39	4.28	0.17	1.40
J	3.51	4.60	0.18	1.47
K	4.31	1.98	0.04	1.10

of the partition coefficient occurred. Propylene glycol addition did not produce any effect. The percentage of the solute passing through the skin from the system correlated well with the partition coefficient, indicating that the skin/system partition coefficient determined the flux.

H. Nicotinates

Albery and Hadgraft[80,81] reported the results of experiments in which the percutaneous absorption of three different esters of nicotinic acid were studied in vivo. These compounds readily penetrate the skin and after several minutes produce a noticeable erythema. Many workers[82,83,89] have found that for the same conditions the time of onset of erythema is reproducible. The erythema is triggered by the direct action of the esters on the blood vessel walls at the junction between the dermis and the epidermis.[85] The time for erythema to be

Table 12
INFLUENCE OF THE PARTITION COEFFICIENT
ON THE PERCUTANEOUS ABSORPTION OF
NICOTINIC ACID AND DERIVATIVES[82]

Compound	Partition coefficient water/ether	Minimum concentration to produce erythema	Penetration index
Nicotinic acid	9.25	1:150	1
Nicotinic acid HCl	45.4	1:150	1
Methyl nicotinate	0.373	1:20,000	133
Ethyl nicotinate	0.136	1:18,000	120
Butyl nicotinate	0.028	1:2,700	18
Hexyl nicotinate	0.012	1:4,000	27
Octyl nicotinate	0.032	1:300	2
Tetrahydrofurfuryl nicotinate	0.394	1:4,300	29

produced has been measured both when the ester is applied continuously and in pulse experiments when the ester is removed before the erythema develops. The results show that the erythema is produced long before steady state diffusion across the epidermis is established.

Results using glycerol-water mixtures in the external phase show that the route of penetration for methyl nicotinate is through the interstitial channels and not through the keratinized cells. Data on the absorption of some other permeants was also found to fit the interstitial route.[67]

Guy and Maibach[86] studied the in vivo human absorption of methyl nicotinate. Topical application of a sufficiently concentrated solution of methyl nicotinate elicits, within minutes, an erythematous, vasodilatory response in humans.

Stoughton et al.[82] showed how the water/ether partition coefficient affected the percutaneous absorption of nicotinic acid and its various derivatives (Table 12). As the size of the alkyl group on nicotinic acid increased, the water/ether partition coefficient declined and the minimum concentration required to produce erythema also decreased.

Sekura and Scala[57] investigated the ability of alkyl methyl sulfoxides to enhance the penetration of sodium nicotinate. Figure 6 shows the effects of sulfoxide concentration on the penetration of sodium nicotinate through guinea pig skin. The data are in agreement with the data of other workers.[23,87,88]

These results show that concentrations of DMSO in excess of 50% are required to obtain an appreciable permeation enhancement. The higher homologs are active at concentrations as low as 2%, with dramatic increases in the permeability with further increase in the sulfoxide concentration. The capability of the sulfoxides to increase the penetration of sodium nicotinate appears to parallel their own ability to penetrate the skin. The most effective is $C_{10}MSO$, which at 10% is a suspension and increases the penetration of nicotinate 55 times. With a slurry of $C_{12}MSO$ at 10%, the skin permeability increases two times, and in a slurry of $C_{14}MSO$ at 10% concentration no apparent increase was observed. A similar result has been reported for the increase of water penetration through rat skin by sodium salts of fatty acids.[89] In the homologous series of fatty acid salts the ten carbon compound was most effective.

I. Phenolic Compounds

Phenolic compounds are weak organic acids which are widely used in topical preparations for their local anesthetic, antipuritic, or antibacterial properties. Under certain conditions, phenol is known to damage skin leading to increased penetration rates.[90,91]

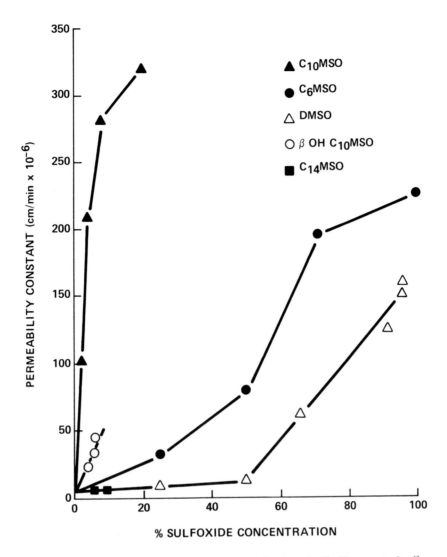

FIGURE 6. Penetration of sodium nicotinate as a function of sulfoxide concentration.[57]

Roberts et al.[92] examined the influence of concentration and chemical structure of various phenolic compounds on the permeability of human skin. The permeability coefficients, threshold concentrations for damage, solubility and partition coefficients are listed in Table 13 (also see References 93-95). The permeation, to a large extent, follows the octanol/water partition coefficient of the particular phenolic compound. The lag times of phenolic compounds differ markedly (Table 14). Phenol, the cresols, and bromophenol have lag times of about 15 min while those for β-naphthol, *m*-nitrophenol, and resorcinol are greater by factors of about 2, 3, and 5, respectively.

The addition of polar groups to a solute decreases its diffusion coefficient in the stratum corneum.[38,96] The longer lag times may be attributed to this effect.

It is suggested that the increased permeability of the stratum corneum above the threshold concentration is caused by damage to the membrane and not by increased activity coefficients for the solutes in the higher concentrations. This conclusion is supported by findings that there is no increase in the permeability at higher concentrations of phenol for permeation through a polyethylene membrane and that the partition coefficient of phenol between arachis oil and water is independent of concentration up to saturation. The differences in flux of

Table 13
PERMEABILITY COEFFICIENTS (I, cm/min × 10^4), THRESHOLD CONCENTRATIONS FOR DAMAGE[a] (II), SOLUBILITY (III), AND PARTITION DATE FOR VARIOUS PHENOLIC COMPOUNDS[93-95]

Solute	I	II (% w/v)	III (% w/v)	$\log_{10}$ P[b]
Resorcinol	0.04	n[c]		0.8
p-Nitrophenol	0.93	0.9	1.4	1.96
m-Nitrophenol	0.94	0.8	1.3	2.00
Phenol	1.37	1.5	7.8	1.46
Methyl hydroxy-benzoate	1.52	n	0.2	1.96
m-Cresol	2.54	1.0	2.5	1.96
o-Cresol	2.62	0.9	2.5	1.96
p-Cresol	2.92	8.85	2.1	1.95
β-Naphthol	4.65	n	0.1	2.84
o-Chlorophenol	5.51	0.8	2.2	2.15
p-Ethylphenol	5.81	n	0.5	2.40
3,4-Xylenol	6.00	n	0.5	2.35
p-Bromophenol	6.02	0.95	1.5	2.59
p-Chlorophenol	6.05	0.75	2.4	2.39
Thymol	8.80	n	0.1	3.34
Chlorocresol	9.16	n	0.5	3.10
Chloroxylenol	9.84	n	0.03	3.39
2,4,6-Trichloro phenol	9.90	n	0.09	3.69
2,4-Dichlorophenol	10.01	n	0.5	3.08

[a] n indicates no damage observed for any concentration of solute up to saturation.
[b] P is the octanol-water partition coefficient of solute.
[c] n indicates no damage up to 40% w/v.

Table 14
LAG TIMES FOR PERMEABILITY EXPERIMENTS[92]

Solute	Concentration (% w/v)	Time lag (min)
Phenol	0.4	15
o-Cresol	0.4	15
m-Cresol	0.4	15
p-Bromophenol	0.4	15
p-Cresol	0.4	16
3,4-Xylenol	0.2	16
Chlorocresol	0.4	17
Chloroxylenol	0.01	18
Thymol	0.10	18
β-Naphthol	0.05	30
m-Nitrophenol	0.5	50
Resorcinol	10	80

Table 15
COMPARISON OF PERMEABILITY
COEFFICIENTS (k_p) OF PENETRANT
FROM A DILUTE AQUEOUS SOLUTION
FOLLOWING CONTACT WITH A
CONCENTRATED SOLUTION[92]

Solute conc used to cause damage	k_p (cm/min × 10^4)		
	Dilute soln	Conc soln	Dilute soln after conc soln
Phenol (5% w/v)	1.1	2.1	2.4
Phenol (s.s.)	1.1	3.3	3.5
p-Nitrophenol (s.s.)	1.2	1.8	1.8
m-Cresol (s.s.)	2.0	3.7	3.4
o-Chlorophenol (s.s.)	3.2	5.0	3.8
p-Chlorophenol (s.s.)	3.5	5.3	4.0
p-Bromophenol (s.s.)	5.6	8.4	7.0

Note: s.s. = saturated solution.

phenol from low concentrations of phenol through excised skin before and after treatment with damaging concentration (Table 15)[92] confirms this effect.

The effect of temperature on the permeation of phenolic compounds from aqueous solution through excised human skin has been examined.[99] From a thermodynamic analysis of the data, a mechanism has been postulated by which the more polar solutes penetrate through human skin. It is suggested that the main resistance to penetration is the lipid barriers in the stratum corneum. Diffusion of these substances through the stratum corneum appears to depend on the breaking of hydrogen bonds in the desolvation of the solute during this penetration process and by the overall viscosity of the stratum corneum. With nonpolar solutes, the aqueous boundary layer appears to provide an additional barrier to the penetration of phenolic compounds.

Recently, Behl et al.[97,98] studied the permeability of phenol through excised hairless mouse skin using normal as well as burn-traumatized skin samples. The permeability results indicate that the hairless mouse is a good model for the human skin. The magnitudes of the permeability coefficients, lag times, concentration effects, and the stripping influences were found to be comparable to those reported earlier for the human skin.

J. Salicylic Acid and Salicylates

Salicylic acid is widely used as a keratolytic and antiseptic agent. The percutaneous absorption of salicylates has been reported extensively[100-106] Barry et al.[106] examined blood salicylate levels in rabbits treated with 10% salicylic acid in hydrophilic ointment at weekly intervals. They reported that a progressive and statistical decrease in the percutaneous absorption of salicylic acid occurred over the treatment period.

Roberts and Horlock[101] applied various concentrations of salicylic acid in hydrophilic ointment repeatedly at daily or weekly intervals to rats in vivo. Salicylic acid absorption through treated skin was monitored by determining the penetration fluxes of salicylic acid through skin excised at various times. Table 16 shows the mean penetration fluxes observed through dimethylpolysiloxane and excised skin along with the ratio of the fluxes. The ratio of fluxes decreased with increasing concentrations of salicylic acid. This result may be ascribed to the suspended salicylic acid particles reducing the occlusive properties of the hydrophilic ointment or to a dehydrating effect of the salicylic acid.

Table 16
MEAN PENETRATION FLUXES (± SE) OF
SALICYLIC ACID IN HYDROPHILIC OINTMENT
BASE THROUGH DIMETHYL POLYSILOXANE
MEMBRANES AND EXCISED RAT SKIN
FOLLOWING A SINGLE TREATMENT[101]

Salicylic acid conc (w/w)	Penetration flux of salicylic acid (±SE), mg/cm²/hr		Ratio of fluxes: skin-dimethyl polysiloxane
	Excised skin	Dimethyl polysiloxane	
1	0.014 ± 0.002	0.016 ± 0.001	0.88
5	0.061 ± 0.003	0.099 ± 0.001	0.62
10	0.078 ± 0.003	0.159 ± 0.001	0.49

Table 17
RELATION BETWEEN ABSORPTION AND
PARTITION COEFFICIENTS OF SALICYLIC ACID
AND CARBINOXAMINE[107]

Salicylic Acid

pH	F. U. F.[a] (%)	Percent absorbed (1-6 hr)	Partition coefficient (at 32°)		
			CHCl₂	Ether	Benzene
2	90.9	6.1 ± 0.6[b]	3.74	>100	0.135
3	50.0	3.3 ± 0.5	1.89	49.5	0.061
4	9.09	0.6 ± 0.2	0.35	13.0	0.006
5	0.99	0	0.04	1.6	0.004

Carbinoxamine

pH	F. U. F. (%)	Percent absorbed (1-6 hr)	Partition coefficient (at 32°)		
			CHCl₂	Ether	Benzene
7	1.2	0	>100	2.7	1.4
8	11.2	1.8 ± 0.6	>100	17.3	7.8
9	55.7	8.0 ± 1.0	>100	95.9	66.8
10	92.6	15.5 ± 1.8	>100	>100	>100

[a]   Fraction of unionized form of the drug.
[b]   Mean ± SD.

Arita et al.[107] studied the relationship of the permeability and partition coefficients of salicylic acid and carbinoxamine, the antihistamine, through intact guinea pig skin (Table 17). The data indicate that there is preferential absorption of the unionized form of the drug.

Elias et al.[108] compared the penetration of water and salicylic acid across abdominal and leg stratum corneum (Table 18). Leg stratum corneum was about two times more permeable than abdominal stratum corneum to water and slightly more permeable to salicylic acid.

Shen et al.[109] studied the effects of 15 nonionic surfactants on the percutaneous absorption of salicylic acid in white petrolatum containing DMSO. They found that the plasma salicylate levels in rabbits were increased significantly when sorbitan trioleate, sorbitan monopalmitate, poloxamer 231, poloxamer 182, polyoxyethylene-4-lauryl-ether, poly-oxyethylene-2-oleyl-

Table 18
PENETRATION OF WATER AND
SALICYLIC ACID ACROSS
ABDOMINAL AND LEG STRATUM
CORNEUM[108]

	Penetration ($\pm$ SEM)	
	Water ($\mu M/cm^2/24$ hr)	Salicylic acid ($\mu M/cm^2/24$ hr)
Abdominal skin	5.4 ± 1.7	4.9 ± 0.4
	2.77 (1 exp.)	3.7 (1 exp.)
	1.95 ± 0.63	0.7 (1 exp.)
	5.47 ± 0.81	9.7 ± 7.8
	1.77 ± 0.34	1.2 ± 0.6
	2.03 ± 0.48	1.4 ± 0.8
	3.2 ± 0.8	3.6 ± 0.6
Leg skin	10.7 ± 3.9	8.7 ± 1.9
	12.7 ± 4.67	7.9 ± 1.8
	4.5 ± 1.2	1.9 ± 0.4
	5.5 ± 1.86	6.8 ± 4.1
	7.6 ± 1.7	5.0 ± 0.8
	7.6 ± 2.15	4.1 ± 1.9
	8.1 ± 2.6	5.7 ± 1.8

ether, or polyoxyl-8-stearate was added to the ointment (Table 19). The mechanism by which the percutaneous absorption of salicylic acid is increased by nonionic surfactants in the presence of DMSO is unknown. However, Higuchi[110] suggested that the activity coefficient of the acid and salt plays a major role in determining the percutaneous absorption. Salicylic acid held firmly by the white petrolatum, forms a drug-vehicle complex exhibiting a low activity coefficient. The rate of release from such drug-vehicle combinations is slow. When DMSO and surfactants are added to the ointment containing 10% (w/w) salicylic acid in white petrolatum, the rate of release of salicylic acid may be increased by forming high activity coefficient complexes such as surfactant-drug, DMSO-drug, and DMSO-surfactant-drug. Therefore, the percutaneous absorption of salicylic acid may be enhanced by these complexes.

Maruta[111] studied the percutaneous absorption of methyl salicylate from a "plaster" applied to the back of the hairless mouse. The peak level (1.5 mg%) of salicylate in the serum was obtained 2 hr after application. Approximately 40% of the dose applied was excreted in the urine of 48-hour treated mice. The same investigator applied sheets of the plaster to the back of male human subjects for 12 hr. The amount absorbed was established to be about 37% of the applied dose. The serum concentrations of total salicylates and free salicylic acid reached a peak at 8 to 12 hr. Within 12 hr after removal of the plaster, practically all of the total salicylates and free salicylic acid were excreted from the body. Application of the plaster for 12 hr a day was repeated for 6 days. Trace or no amount of total salicylates and free salicylic acid were detected in the serum 12 and 36 hr after removal of the last plasters. No significant changes were noted in hepatic function before and after the repeated application.

K. Acetyl Salicylic Acid

Bronaugh[12] compared the percutaneous absorption of acetyl salicylic acid in vivo and in

Table 19

t-TEST VALUE FROM THE COMPARISON OF THE OVERALL AVERAGE OF PERCUTANEOUS SALICYLATE ABSORPTION FROM THE RABBIT BETWEEN SURFACTANT (S) PLUS SALICYLIC ACID (I) PLUS WHITE PETROLATUM USP (II) AND SALICYLIC ACID PLUS WHITE PETROLATUM USP OINTMENTS AND ALSO BETWEEN DMSO (III) PLUS SALICYLIC ACID PLUS WHITE PETROLATUM USP AND DIMETHYL SULFOXIDE PLUS SURFACTANT PLUS SALICYLIC ACID PLUS WHITE PETROLATUM USP OINTMENTS[109]

Surfactant	t-Value between I + II and S + I + II	t-Value between III + S + I + II and III + I + II
Poloxamer 231	4.905[a]	3.886[a]
Poloxamer 182	4.050[a]	5.737[a]
Poloxamer 184	2.992[a]	2.960[a]
Polyoxyethylene 20 oleyl ether	2.461[a]	2.112[a]
Polyoxyethylene 4 lauryl ether	3.154[a]	2.944[a]
Polyoxyethylene 2 oleyl ether	5.918[a]	3.245[a]
Sorbitan monolaurate	3.038[a]	4.537[a]
Sorbitan monopalmitate	11.308[a]	9.877[a]
Sorbitan trioleate	5.435[a]	9.014[a]
Polysorbate 20	2.104[a]	1.165[b]
Polysorbate 40	2.385[a]	0.745[b]
Polysorbate 60	2.886[a]	0.937[b]
Polyoxyl 8 stearate	2.815[a]	3.972[a]
Polyoxyethylene 30 monostearate	1.901[a]	2.164[a]
Polyoxyethylene 40 monostearate	1.851[a]	3.669[a]
Sorbitan trioleate plus polysorbate 40	3.784[a]	3.804[a]
Polyoxyethylene 20 oleyl ether plus polyoxyethylene2 oleyl ether	4.846[a]	4.226[a]
Polyoxyl 8 stearate plus polyoxyethylene 40 monostearate	3.380[a]	3.879[a]

[a] Significant difference at 95% level.
[b] No significant difference.

Table 20
PERCUTANEOUS
ABSORPTION OF
ACETYLSALICYLIC ACID
IN RATS[a][12]

Days	Absorption (% of applied dose)	
	In vivo	**In vitro**
1	8.5 ± 1.6	8.8 ± 1.2
2	7.9 ± 2.0	8.5 ± 1.2
3	4.0 ± 0.9	4.6 ± 0.5
4	2.8 ± 0.5	4.3 ± 0.4
5	1.9 ± 0.5	2.9 ± 0.1
Total	24.8 ± 4.4	29.0 ± 3.1

[a]   Results are expressed as the $\bar{x}$ of SE
of four or five determinations.

vitro using rat skin (Table 20). The values of 24.8 and 29.0% absorbed of the applied dose
show good correlation. These values compare favorably to the 21.8% value obtained by
Feldman and Maibach in humans,[112] but not to the 40.5% value which Franz[11] reported.

Loftson and Bodor[113] investigated the topical permeation of the sulfoxide and sulphone
prodrug derivatives of aspirin through the hairless mouse skin. The methylthiomethyl and
methylsulfinylmethyl-2-acetoxybenzoate penetrate freshly excised hairless mouse skin rather
easily with the simultaneous hydrolysis of the two ester functions. Contrary to in vivo
observations in dogs, where significant amounts of aspirin formed, the prodrugs cleave to
salicylic acid and/or salicylate esters rather than aspirin. The permeability coefficients and
lag times of these compounds are listed in Table 21. The methylthiomethyl derivative of
aspirin is absorbed at a rate about two times faster than that of aspirin, while the methylsulfinylmethyl derivative is absorbed at the same rate as aspirin within the experimental
error. The amounts penetrating the skin, however, are significant.

L. Iodochlorohydroxyquin

Iodochlorohydroxyquin (Clioquinol, Vioform), an antifungal agent, is used in the treatment
of diaper rash and other skin disorders and was presumed to undergo little or no percutaneous
absorption. However, three relatively recent studies have demonstrated significant percutaneous absorption.[114-116] Stohs et al.[116] studied the absorption from a 3% cream in normal
male subjects after a single application of the cream for 12 hr. Plasma levels of the drug
were followed for 24 hr after initial application while urinary excretion was measured for
54 hr. The drug in the range of 0.37 to 0.56 μg/mℓ was detected in plasma 2 hr after
application but could not be detected within 1 hr. A steady-state level was reached at
approximately 4 hr. Although the remaining topically applied drug was removed after 12
hr, plasma levels were still elevated 24 hr after initial application. The mean excretion rate
after 12 hr of application was 58.4 μg/hr and the rate was 8.8 μg/hr at 42-hr post treatment.
The elimination rate constant was calculated to be 0.5/hr. Approximately 40% of the drug
was absorbed over the 12-hr application period.

Fischer and Hartvig[114] found that after treatment with Vioform-Locorten (glucocorticoid)
cream (15 to 20 g over 40% body area, twice daily, corresponding to 1.2 g clioquinol/day)
the urinary excretion was 3 to 4% of the dose. The same authors reported the application
of Locacorten-Vioform cream and/or ointment to patients with various skin diseases. About
30 to 70% of the body area was treated with daily amounts of cream or ointment corresponding

Table 21
**PERMEABILITY COEFFICIENT AND LAG
TIMES FOR APPARENT PERMEABILITY OF
ASPIRIN AND METHYLTHIOMETHYL AND
METHYLSULFINYLMETHYL 2-
ACETOXYBENZOATES THROUGH EXCISED
HAIRLESS MICE SKIN AT 31°C** [113]

Compound applied	Compound detected in receptor phase[a]	Permeability coefficient (cm/hr)	Lag time (hr)
Aspirin	I	$4.9 \pm 1.0 \times 10^{-3}$	0.82
	II	$1.4 \pm 0.1 \times 10^{-2}$	0.72
	Total	$1.9 \pm 0.2 \times 10^{-2}$	0.77
III	II	$4.0 \pm 0.5 \times 10^{-2}$	0.70
IV	V	$9.6 \pm 4.0 \times 10^{-3}$	1.18
	II	$1.2 \pm 0.6 \times 10^{-2}$	0.33
	Total	$2.2 \pm 1.0 \times 10^{-2}$	0.87

Note: Compounds: (I) aspirin, (II) salicylic acid, (III) methylthiomethyl ester, (IV) methylsulfinylmethyl ester, (V)
methylsulfinylmethyl 2-hydroxybenzoate.

[a] The compounds detected in the receptor phase were aspirin
(I), salicylic acid (II), and methylsulfinylmethyl 2-hydrox-
ybenzoate (V).

to 0.48 to 0.98 g clioquinol. The plasma levels of clioquinol rose to 0.3 to 1.3 μg/mℓ within
1 hr after application. Four days after the treatment was stopped, only negligible concentrations of clioquinol were found in the plasma. Urinary excretion of clioquinol was measured
on the fourth day of the treatment and found to amount to 2.2 to 7.5% of the applied dose.
Of the total excreted amount, 95% consisted of conjugated metabolites. Noticeable is the
fact that even when applying large amounts of clioquinol containing creams into the diseased
skins, the percent absorption is in the same range as found after administration on healthy
skins in this study.

Degen et al.[115] obtained similar results. In their studies, Vioform cream, Locacorten-
Vioform cream, and Vioform-Hydrocortisone cream in amounts containing 30 mg clioquinol
were applied under occlusive dressings to the healthy skin of volunteers. On average, 2.5%
of the dose was excreted in urine. Among the different topical preparations, no distinct
differences in the excretion pattern could be observed. On average, about 69% of the total
amount excreted in the urine was eliminated in all volunteers within the first 24 hr. About
9.3% of the dose was excreted in 48-hr postapplication. After oral administration of an equal
dose, the urinary excretion amounted to 52 to 93% of the dose. As in case of the topical
application, main excretion occurred within the first 48 hr.

M. Dithranol

Dithranol (anthralin) is used for the treatment of psoriasis. Kammerau et al.[117] studied
the penetration kinetics of dithranol and triacetyl-dithranol in intact human skin (in vivo).
The penetration of both substances was considerably influenced by the carrier. Lipophilic
ointment bases, particularly the single-phase base petrolatum, allowed the best penetration
of both drugs into the epidermis. The maximal amount penetrating into the epidermis was
0.3 μg/cm^2 of the skin surface for dithranol and 0.04 μg/cm^2 for triacetyl-dithranol in

petrolatum. From petrolatum the maximal dermal concentrations were in a reversed relationship: 0.1 $\mu g/cm^2$ for triacetyl-dithranol and 0.045 $\mu g/cm^2$ for dithranol.

From hydrophilic ointments, only poor penetration was observed; about 0.1 $\mu g/cm^2$ of triacetyl-dithranol into the epidermis. The application of a hydrophilic single-phase base brings about a high depot in the horny layer for both substances. The data indicate that the triacetate was not split into its parent compound, dithranol, in substantial quantity. The data obtained show the criteria of two independent substances.

If the free hydrophilic groups of dithranol are blocked, e.g., esterified with acetic acid in triacetyl-dithranol, then, as expected, the physicochemical properties of dithranol are altered and as a consequence the extremely rapid penetration through the human skin is lost.[117] There is no reason to assume the active transport in the skin. The fact that the concentrations of dithranol in the epidermis are higher than in the horny layer therefore reflects very clearly different physicochemical properties of these two layers. A partition of the drug between two phases takes place where one phase, the epidermal tissue, has a far greater affinity for the substance than does the horny layer. Together with the reduced barrier function of the horny layer, this behavior indicates a considerably high absorption rate of dithranol.

Selim[118] and Schalla[119] carried out in vitro investigations of the penetration of anthralin into human skin. Selim[118] noted that the drug penetrates the skin and attains the highest concentration in the upper part of the epidermis. The drug is probably conjugated and is concentrated within the cells around the nuclei with a sharp decrease in the gradient in the lower epidermis and corium. The penetration of the drug in vitro takes place shortly after application and the distribution becomes stabilized so that there is little difference between 1 and 24 hr of application. Schalla[119] noted that the barrier function is not so pronounced as with the other drugs. Removal of the horny layer enhanced the influx by a factor of 2.3. For most other substances investigated, the influx increases in the range of five to tenfold. The urinary excretion, which is continued over a long period after a single topical application, is rate limited by the percutaneous absorption process. Such behavior is well known in other compounds and indicates a reservoir, as with anthralin, which is at least partially located in the horny layer.

N. Xanthines

1. Caffeine

Zesch et al.[120] studied the distribution of caffeine in the skin layers after topical application from varied ointment bases (Table 22). The caffeine is rapidly taken up in the epidermis and corium in continuously increasing quantities until a maximum is attained after 100 min. A penetrating time of 300 min brings about a distinct decrease in the quantities penetrating in the epidermis and corium.

Best penetration into the horny layer after 100 min was from the w/o wool wax (2.182 $\mu g/cm^2$) and least well from the polyethylene glycol ointment (0.632 $\mu g/cm^2$). The o/w emulsion provided the best penetration of the barrier and relatively high concentrations in the epidermis (0.508 $\mu g/cm^2$). The single phase ointment bases, vaseline, and polyethylene glycol behave similarly, with penetration of 0.204 and 0.216 $\mu g/cm^2$, respectively. The lowest quantity penetrating into the epidermis (0.137 $\mu g/cm^2$) is found with w/o emulsions. It should be noted that the highest levels of this substance are found after this 100-min penetration period, rather than the other times employed. Using the o/w emulsions with which high epidermal concentrations were attained, the greatest quantity penetrates into the corium (0.667 $\mu g/cm^2$). The lowest levels are attained (0.056 $\mu g/cm^2$) with the w/o emulsion. Vaseline and polyethylene glycol ointments result in similar values (0.090 and 0.108 $\mu g/cm^2$, respectively). It appears, therefore, that the quantities of substance found in the corium are proportional in all cases to those found in the epidermis. The purine derivative penetrates

Table 22
IN VITRO LEVELS, EXPRESSED AS μg SUBSTANCE/CM²
SURFACE APPLIED IN RELATION TO THE OINTMENT
BASE AND PERIOD OF PENETRATION OF CAFFEINE[120]

Skin layer	Penetration time (min)	Vaseline	Aqueous woolwax alcohol ointment	Aqueous hydrophilic ointment	Polyethylene glycol ointment
Horny layer	10	0.659	0.643	1.491	0.845
	30	1.358	1.464	1.978	0.832
	100	1.527	2.182	1.542	0.632
	300	2.362	1.592	2.362	0.797
	1000	1.550	2.326	1.550	0.081
Epidermis	10	0.012	0.019	0.133	0.001
	30	0.016	0.008	0.042	0.052
	100	0.204	0.137	0.508	0.216
	300	0.023	0.064	0.023	0.039
	1000	0.105	0.246	0.105	0.049
Corium	10	0.005	0.010	0.022	0.001
	30	0.028	0.009	0.215	0.007
	100	0.090	0.056	0.667	0.109
	300	0.072	0.144	0.072	0.037
	1000	0.306	0.450	0.306	0.072

from o/w emulsion over brief application periods at 100-fold higher levels than steroids into the epidermis.

Feldman and Maibach[112] reported about 48% of the applied topical dose of caffeine is found in the urine following application from an acetone solution.

2. Theophylline

Xanthines, such as theophylline, modify adenosine-3′5′-monophosphate-cAMP response. The hypothesis that cAMP and cAMP-modifying agents mediate inflammatory responses and the suggestion that low levels of cAMP were somehow responsible for psoriasis have led to numerous attempts to treat various inflammatory conditions and psoriasis with agents known to affect cAMP levels. Theophylline is typical of many such agents, but has only a narrow therapeutic range in the oral treatment of asthma. Thus, doses of theophylline that would be high enough to regulate cAMP also would result in blood levels that are very close to systemic toxic levels. The ideal solution to the problem of the narrow systemic therapeutic range would be to deliver theophylline topically for the treatment of psoriasis. This would eliminate the necessity of high systemic levels of theophylline and would result in local therapeutically effective levels. However, theophylline is a high melting, polar, lipophobic molecule which hinders its facile absorption through the skin.[110]

Sloan and Bodor[121] studied the topical penetration of a series of 7-acyloxymethyl prodrugs of theophylline through excised hairless mouse skin. Table 23 shows the structures of the theophylline prodrugs and the results of the diffusion experiments. The lipid solubilities of all the prodrugs were markedly improved over that of theophylline. Structures III and IV were 3.5 and 4.4 times more effective than theophylline at delivering theophylline through skin from an isopropyl myristate vehicle. 7-(Hydroxymethyl) theophylline was also quite effective at delivering theophylline topically; almost five times as effective as theophylline.

The lag time (1.7 hr) for theophylline, III, and IV are all the same but the lag time for II is apparently much longer (4.3 hr) and it exhibits an apparently greater rate of delivery of I, just the opposite of what would normally be expected from the relative lag time. The greater rate of delivery of I by II appears to be primarily a consequence of II being 16 times

Table 23
DIFFUSION OF THEOPHYLLINE AND ITS PRODRUGS THROUGH HAIRLESS MOUSE SKIN[121]

	Compound	%Conc[a]	Mole of applied drug in soln ($\times 10^6$)[b]	% of applied drug as theophylline diffused after 12 hr	Mole of applied drug as theophylline diffused after 12 hr ($\times 10^6$) mean ± SD[c]
I	R = H	6.5	0.067	4.5	4.81 ± 0.35
II	R = CH_2OH	7.5	1.05	22.3	23.59 ± 5.96[d]
V	R = $CH_2O_2CC_3H_7$	10.0	9.0	19.9	21.41 ± 2.19[d]
VIII	R = $CH_2O_2CC(CH_3)_3$	10.5	6.75	16.0[e]	16.97 ± 2.68[d,e]

[a]   Total drug in suspension and solution.
[b]   Average of 3 determinations ± <1% in isopropyl myristate.
[c]   n = 3.
[d]   The rate of delivery of I by II (6.16 × 10⁻⁷ ± 1.66 × 10⁻⁷ mol/cm² · hr) was significantly different ($p < 0.05$) from the rate of delivery of I by V (4.03 × 10⁻⁷ ± 3.54 × 10⁻⁹ mol/cm² · hr) and the rate of delivery of I by VIII (3.3 × 10⁻⁷ ± 5.1 × 10⁻⁹ mol/cm² · hr) was significantly different ($p < 0.05$) from the rate of delivery of I by V based on the mean ± S.D. of the slopes of lines in Figure 1.
[e]   Contains 14.5 ± 5% of the theophylline as intact VIII.

more soluble than I in isopropyl myristate.[110,112] Thus, although the acyloxymethyl prodrug approach has not been optimized, it has been shown that 7-acyloxymethyl derivatives of theophylline are, indeed, prodrugs which effectively increase the delivery of theophylline through the skin and that once the theophylline has been delivered, it is an effective antiproliferative agent.

O. Organophosphates (Sarin)

Wurster et al.[123] studied the permeability of the nerve gas, Sarin, isopropoxymethylphosphoryl fluoridate, across excised human skin. The average Sarin transport rates through callus membranes for each experimental series are given in Table 24. The results show that interaction between the membrane and penetrant plays a significant role in Sarin transport across human skin.

The same group continued the study of determining the effect of solvent pretreatment of callus membranes with DMSO, dimethylacetamide, dimethyl formamide, formamide, dioxane, and methyl orthoformate on Sarin transport rates.[124] The permeability coefficients at each temperature and activation energy for each system are shown in Table 25, with the expected inverse order between the rate ratio and the activation energy being observed. Pretreatment with formamide and dimethylsulfoxide appreciably increased the permeability coefficients. Dioxane and methyl orthoformate caused only slight increases.

P. Steroids

Steroids constitute the single most studied class of compounds whose percutaneous absorption characteristics have been extensively studied. In several studies,[32,125,126] in general,

Table 24
AVERAGE TRANSPORT RATES OF SARIN ACROSS CALLUS TISSUE MEMBRANES FOR VARIOUS SYSTEMS[123]

Experimental conditions	Transport rate (mg/cm²/hr)
Sarin in *n*-heptane, anhydrous membrane	0.03
Pure sarin, anhydrous membrane	0.60
8% Polymethyl methacrylate gel, anhydrous membrane	0.49
3% Carboxypolymethylene gel, anhydrous membrane	0.55
8% Polymethyl methacrylate gel, hydrous membrane	1.1
3% Carboxypolymethylene gel, hydrous membrane	2.76

Table 25
PERMEABILITY COEFFICIENTS AND ACTIVATION ENERGIES FOR SOLVENT-TREATED MEMBRANES[124]

Membrane conditioning solvent	Temperature (°C)	Permeability coefficient ($K \times 10^4$/hr)	Activation energy (kcal/mol)
DMSO	24.9	13.00	8.2
	35.0	18.65	
	44.9	31.09	
Dioxane	25.0	4.13	21.2
	34.9	11.72	
	44.9	39.00	
Methyl orthoformate	25.0	2.75	22.3
	34.9	10.05	
	44.8	28.79	
Dimethylformamide	26.0	1.07	14.4
	35.1	1.83	
	45.0	4.54	
Formamide	25.0	28.29	6.2
	35.0	37.51	
	44.5	54.16	

the chemical structure did not appear to influence the rate of absorption, but Scheuplein and co-workers[96] showed that is has some relevance in the absorption of steroids. Table 26 contains a summary of the human permeability coefficients of various steroids.[96] These data were computed from the steady-state flux-time curves. Steroids were chosen because they provided a wide range in polarity within restricted limits of molecular weight. A 1000-fold difference in the permeabilities of estrone to hydrocortisone cannot be explained only on a difference between their molecular weights which differ by about 25%.

The large differences observed in the permeabilities of these steroids can be apportioned between the solubility of the steroids within the membrane and their diffusivities through it. The solubility in the stratum corneum can, however, explain only a small part of the observed permeability. Table 26 shows that the partition coefficient changes much less than the permeability coefficient. It can be seen from the tabulated data that the lower permeabilities of the polar steroids do not arise from a limited solubility within the membrane but from their decreased molecular mobility due to stronger chemical binding. The major factor responsible for decreasing the permeability of the steroids over that of smaller molecules is

Table 26
PERMEABILITY COEFFICIENTS AND RELATED
DATA FOR STEROIDS[96]

Steroid	$\Delta Cs \times 10^9$ mol/mℓ	$P \times 10^6$ (cm/hr)	$D \times 10^3$ cm^2/sec	Km
Progesterone	2.0	1500	160	104
Pregnenolone	5.1	1500	220	50
Hydroxypregnenolone	2.9	600	155	43
Hydroxyprogasterone	10.0	600	166	40
Cortexone	2.4	450	135	37
Testosterone	10.0	400	195	23
Cortexolone	10.0	75	36.1	23
Corticosterone	1.7	60	39.2	17
Cortisone	1.0	10	13.1	9
Hydrocortisone	1.8	3	4.8	7
Aldosterone	0.7	3	4.9	7
Estrone	2.5	3600	870.0	46
Estradiol	2.5	300	72.4	46
Estriol	7.0	40	19.3	23
Betamethasone valerate	—	6	—	—
Hydrocortisone valerate	—	3	—	—
Hydrocortisone butyrate	—	0.2	—	—

the decrease in the diffusion constant. A 3 to 4 times greater molar volume than that of an average small molecule can partly explain the decreased diffusivity.

Introducing additional polar groups into the steroidal molecules further lowers their diffusion constants. Figure 7 indicates how the steroidal permeability progressively decreases as the compounds become increasingly more polar in going from progesterone to cortisol. Introducing successive hydroxyl groups into the molecule starting with progesterone and going to cortexone, cortexolone, and finally to cortisol leads to a cumulative decrease in both the diffusion and the permeability constants. A similar phenomenon is shown to occur for the estrogen steroids, compounds containing an aromatic A-ring. Such influences complicate the issue and one cannot expect a proportionality between permeability constant and partition coefficient.

In a recent study,[127] 21 esters of hydrocortisone were prepared placing a side chain of varying alkyl length and their permeabilities were determined through the hairless mouse skin. The results indicated an exponential increase in the permeability as a function of the side alkyl chain length (Figure 8). The partition coefficients of these derivatives increase with increasing the alkyl chain length. This is an important observation because it again stresses that the single most important factor determining the skin permeability of a compound is its partition coefficient. Such chemical structure alterations are of practical value because the desired skin permeability can be obtained in this manner if the biological activity of the parent molecule is not affected.

Q. Azo Dyes

The toxicity of azo hair dyes has been of concern. Maibach and Wolfram[166] determined the percutaneous absorption of hair dyes in the rhesus monkey and man. The study design was relevant in that the ^{14}C-labeled materials were incorporated in commercially available hair dye products. Human volunteers received an actual hair-dying procedure. Rhesus monkeys were similarly treated (also using the hair on the scalp). Both species showed a remarkably similar pattern of dye penetration. The average dose excretion of diaminoanisole in the rhesus monkey was 0.02 and 0.15% in man; *p*-phenylenediamine excretion in monkey

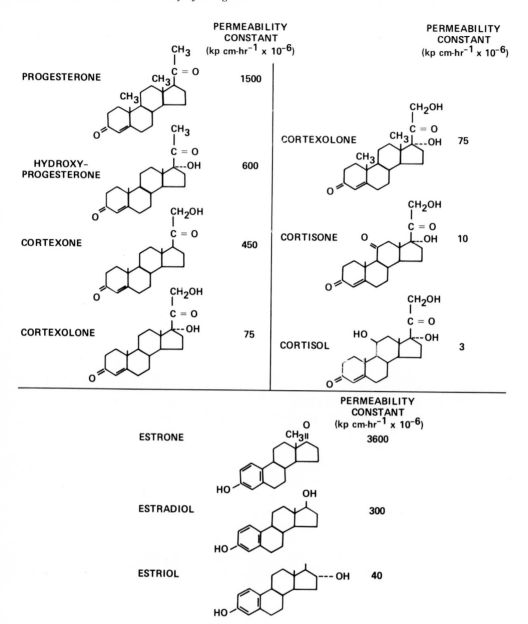

FIGURE 7.   Permeability constants of an homologous group of steroids. The molecules are made increasingly more polar by the introduction of carbonyl and hydroxyl groups.[96]

and man was 0.14% and HC Blue #1 excretion in monkey was 0.12% and in man was 0.09%. Marzulli[128] measured the skin penetration of 2,4-toluenediamine (2,4 TDA), 2,4-diaminoanisole (2,4-DAA, also known as 4-methoxy-*m*-phenylenediamine or 4-MMPD), and 2-nitro-*p*-phenylenediamine (NPPD) in vitro in humans, monkeys, and swine. The greatest skin penetration was recorded with 2,4-toluenediamine applied to the abdominal skin of monkeys and the least with 2,4-diaminoanisole on the monkey abdomen and human ventral forearm. 2-Nitro-*p*-phenylenediamine showed intermediate degrees of skin penetration.

Bronaugh[68] determined the partition coefficients and permeability constants of five dyes. They are listed in Table 27 in the order of increasing octanol/water partition coefficient. With the apparent exception of the last compound, this is also the order of increasing

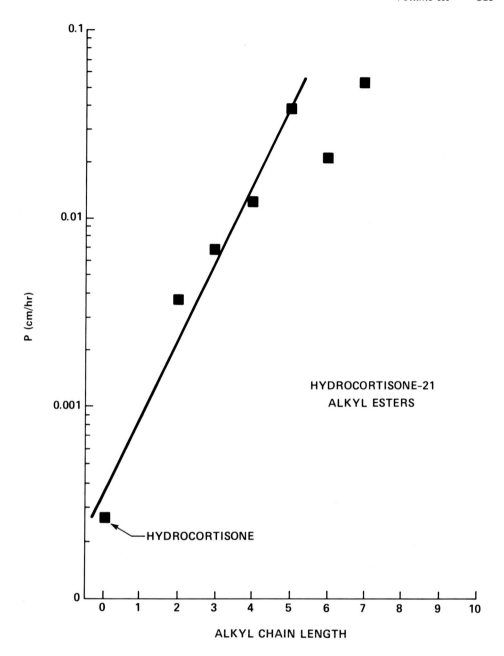

FIGURE 8. Effect of alkyl chain length derivatization on the hairless mouse skin permeability of hydrocortisone.[127]

permeability. Unlike the other dyes, 2-amino-4-nitrophenol is ionized at pH 9.7 and penetrates skin at a rate below the detection limits. When this compound was tested from a water vehicle (dye unionized), penetration was much faster as the partition coefficient would predict. A hair dye predominantly in the ionized form would therefore be much less readily absorbed across the skin barrier. It appears that the effect on skin permeation of alterations in the functional groups on the benzene ring is determined by the net effect on the octanol/water partition coefficient of the molecule.

R. Surface Active Agents

Surface active agents differ considerably in their ability to penetrate the epidermal barrier,

Table 27
PERCUTANEOUS ABSORPTION OF HAIR DYES[68]

Compound	Structure	Octanol/water partition coefficient	Permeability constant (cm/hr)[a]
p-Phenylenediamine		0.5	2.4×10^{-4}
o-Phenylenediamine			
2-Nitro-p-phenylenediamine		2.2	4.5×10^{-4}
2-Amino-4-nitrophenol		3.4	5.0×10^{-4}
4-Chloro-m-phenylenediamine		13.5	$<3.0 \times 10^{-5}$ (6.6×10^{-4})
		7.0	2.1×10^{-3}

[a]   Values were obtained with a borate buffer pH 9.7 as the vehicle, except the number in parentheses, which was obtained in water to prevent ionization.

at least when low concentrations are involved. They can alter the kinetics of drug permeation through the skin by a direct effect on the skin barrier through complexation or solubilization of the drug or by improving wetting of the membrane.[38,89,129-136]

Anionic surfactants penetrate poorly, but prolonged contact or greater concentration increases the permeability of the skin to both detergents themselves and to other substances.[133,137-140] Most in vitro studies were characterized by an extended lag time of several hours whereas, in vivo, a rapid penetration giving measurable blood levels at 15 min[89] and a deeper penetration into skin were recorded. After an initial lag time, the permeability of the skin increases with respect to time. This means that the barrier to penetration decreases during the time the surfactant is in contact with the skin. Cationic surfactants show approximately the same magnitude of permeation as the anionics.[131,139]

The penetration of sodium laurate and sodium dodecyl sulfate (SDS) was investigated by Blank and Gould[133] on excised human abdominal skin. They found that 20 hr after application, sodium laurate had penetrated the epidermis and dermis from weak (0.005 *M*) unbuffered, mildly alkaline aqueous solutions. SDS (0.005 *M*), on the other hand, had penetrated only in very small quantities below the barrier and for the most part was retained in the stratum corneum. This difference was attributed to a greater affinity of the skin proteins to SDS and is in keeping with the observations that alkyl sulfates and alkyl benzene sulfonates combine with proteins to an appreciable extent.[141,142]

Howes[132] measured the permeability constants of a series of anionic surfactants (Table 28) through excised human epidermis. The data confirm the findings of previous workers

Table 28
PERMEABILITY CONSTANTS
(μcm/min) OF SOME ANIONIC
SURFACTANTS THROUGH
ISOLATED HUMAN
EPIDERMIS[132]

Surfactant	Time of contact with surfactant soln (hr)		
	6	24	48
Soaps			
$C_{10:0}$	5.4	18.6	—
$C_{12:0}$	18.2	25.0	—
$C_{14:0}$	1.6	9.4	—
$C_{16:0}$	0.1	0.2	—
$C_{18:0}$	0.1	0.1	—
SDI[a]	0.7	0.9	1.3
SDS[b]	0.1	1.8	35
DOBS[c]	0.1	0.1	—

Note: The sodium soaps were applied as a 6 mM solution in a model soap solution. The SDS and SDI were applied as 25 mM solutions and the DOBS as a 3 mM aqueous solution.

[a] Sodium dodecyl sulfate.
[b] Sodium dodecyl isethionate.
[c] Sodium dodecylbenzenesulphonate.

that the $C_{12:0}$ soap (sodium laurate) penetrates isolated human epidermis most readily of the soaps.[130,135] The increasing rate of penetration of the surfactants during prolonged application was also confirmed. The penetration of sodium dodecyl isethionate (SDI) through human epidermis in vitro gave a penetration rate curve similar to that obtained with the soaps, but SDS showed a long lag time (6 hr) before any penetration occurred after which time the rate of penetration rapidly increased.

Nonionic surfactants generally have little effect in promoting percutaneous absorption. Of the various surfactant classes, the nonionics have the least tendency to interact with the skin barrier and alter membrane permeability.[28,38,100,109,122,129,136,143-147]

Black and Gupta[148] investigated skin penetration in the rat of the anionic alcohol sulfates and alcohol ether sulfates and the nonionic alcohol ethoxylates. The extent to which the surfactants penetrated rat skin is summarized in Table 29, from which it can be seen that the penetration of the alcohol sulfates and alcohol ether sulfates were similar, and low, whereas that of the alcohol ethoxylates was considerably greater. The nonionic series showed firstly an increased penetration with chain elongation of the parent alcohol, in contrast to the anionics, and secondly a reduction in penetration when ethoxylation was increased beyond six residues.

Nishiyama[148A] studied the in vivo percutaneous absorption of polyoxyethylene lauryl ether (LAEO) surfactants in hairless mice to determine the effect of varying the ethylene oxide chain. The absorption data in Table 30 (Part A) shows that the parent compound, lauryl alcohol and the one mole ethoxylate (LAEO-1) and LAEO-2.6 penetrate the skin readily, while LAEO-10 is barely absorbed. Hence, an increase in ethoxylation decreases penetration. A similar relationship is seen in the absorption rate shown in Table 30, Part B. Lauryl

Table 29
SUMMARY OF RAT SKIN
PENETRATION BY
SURFACTANTS

Surfactant	Penetration (in 48 hr) (μg/cm^2)
$nC_{12}SO_4$	0.26 $\pm$ 0.14 (10)
$nC_{15}SO_4$	0.08 $\pm$ 0.04 (6)
$nC_{12}E_3SO_4$	0.39 $\pm$ 0.12 (3)
$nC_{15}E_3SO_4$	0.26 $\pm$ 0.19 (11)
$nC_{12}E_3$	4.38 $\pm$ 0.54 (3)
$nC_{12}E_6$	4.88 $\pm$ 0.42 (9)
$nC_{12}E_{10}$	0.85 $\pm$ 0.26 (3)
$nC_{15}E_3$	8.3 $\pm$ 4.5 (10)

Note: Penetration figures are mean results $\pm$ SD for the number of rats given in parenthesis and are based on the corrected excretion of radioactivity during 48 hr from animals treated with 1% (w/v) solution of the surfactant in 1% (w/v) LAS.

Table 30
PERCUTANEOUS
ABSORPTION DATA OF
LAURYL ALCOHOL
ETHOXYLATE (LAEO)
SURFACTANTS[148A]

Part A

Sample name	% Absorbed
Lauryl alcohol	46.1 $\pm$ 0.9
LAEO-1	56.1 $\pm$ 4.2
LAEO-2.6	61.2 $\pm$ 2.8
LAEO-6.4	27.8 $\pm$ 2.8
LAEO-10	4.9 $\pm$ 0.4

Part B

LAEO	Rate of percutaneous absorption (μmol/cm$^2 \cdot$ hr)
Lauryl alcohol	12.2 $\times$ 10^{-2}
LAEO-1	9.77 $\times$ 10^{-2}
LAEO-2.6	9.78 $\times$ 10^{-2}
LAEO-10	0.75 $\times$ 10^{-2}

alcohol was the fastest followed by LAEO-2.6 and LAEO-1. LAEO-10 had a slower rate by one order of magnitude.

The data on the skin penetration of surface active agents indicate that they differ considerably in their ability to alter the permeability properties of the skin barrier. Unfortunately, the degree of lowering of the surface tension of water is not always given so that it is impossible to say to what extent this difference is related to the surface active property of the solution. The work of Bettley[149] would suggest that lowering the surface tension of water is not an important factor in enhancing skin permeability despite the possibility of removal of lipids when the surface tension of water is lowered. In vitro observations are obviously necessary before one can be certain on this point. The observations of Blank and Gould[133] and of Sprott[89] would indicate that the protein binding ability of the surfactant and the consequent alteration of the structure of the stratum corneum has to be taken into account as one of the factors that influence the alteration of the permeability of the skin. Later studies[39,144] tend to confirm the importance of protein denaturation in the increased permeability of the skin induced by some surfactants. Surfactants are discussed as penetration enhancers in a later chapter.

Many investigators have measured the effects of surfactants on the transfer of other molecules.[39,89,130,131,135,136,149-151]

Chowhan[143,152] has noted that the anionic surfactants, sodium laurate and sodium lauryl sulfate increased the in vitro flux of naproxen, the anti-inflammatory analgesic.

Aguiar and Weiner[136] studied the absorption of the antibiotic, chloramphenicol through excised hairless mouse skin in the presence of sodium lauryl sulfate and polysorbate 80. The effect of adding sodium lauryl sulfate on the permeation rates of chloramphenicol is summarized in Table 31. At a concentration of 0.2% of the surfactant, which is slightly above the critical micelle concentration, the permeation rate was found to be about twice as fast as that without surfactant. Increasing the concentration of sodium lauryl sulfate to 0.4% increases the rate only slightly more than that seen with the 0.2% concentration.

Table 31
EFFECT OF VARIOUS CONCENTRATIONS OF SODIUM LAURYL SULFATE ON THE PERMEATION RATE OF CHLORAMPHENICOL THROUGH THE HAIRLESS MICE SKIN AT 37°C[136]

Conc. of sodium lauryl sulfate (%)	Permeability coeff. cm/min × 10³
0	0.682
0.02	0.298
0.20	1.252
0.40	1.455

Table 32
EFFECT OF VARIOUS CONCENTRATIONS OF POLYSORBATE 80 ON THE PERMEATION RATE OF CHLORAMPHENICOL THROUGH THE SKIN OF HAIRLESS MICE AT 37°C[136]

Conc. of polysorbate 80 (%)	Permeability coeff. (cm/min)
0	0.682×10^{-2}
0.2	0.609×10^{-2}
0.5	0.757×10^{-2}
1.0	1.048×10^{-2}

Polysorbate 80 (a nonionic surfactant), at a concentration higher than the critical micelle concentration has a similar influence on the permeation of chloramphenicol through the skin, although its effect is not as great as that seen with the sodium lauryl sulfate. The data are summarized in Table 32 which shows a slight decrease in the rate at 0.2% concentration and an increase at the higher concentrations.

Shen et al.[109] found that the percutaneous absorption of salicylic acid and sodium salicylate was increased significantly in the presence of varied nonionic surfactants (see section on salicylates for details).

S. Macromolecules

Higher molecular weight compounds show variable penetration.[153,154] Macromolecules such as colloidal sulfur, albumin, dextrans, polyvinyl pyrrolidone, and polypeptides can penetrate the barrier if applied in solvents which possess a high lipid solubility, although they hardly penetrate at all if applied in an aqueous solvent.

The prime study is by Tregear[153] who measured the rabbit and human skin penetration of serum albumin, polyvinyl pyrrolidone, and two dextrans having molecular weight of 94,000 and 153,000.

The albumin penetrated the intact skin at a slower rate than it penetrated the excised skin. The labeled polyvinyl pyrrolidone penetrated the slowest; the lower molecular weight dextran penetrated the fastest. Very large molecules such as proteins and polysaccharides went through very poorly, if at all. Table 33 compares the permeability to rabbit and human skin of HSA, PVP, and the two dextran fractions. The permeability constant of rabbit skin was, on average, approximately 2 to 3 times that of human skin.

A comparison can be made of the results with the skin penetration of smaller molecules. Many small covalent aqueous solutes have permeability constants through rabbit skin in the region of 20 μcm/min, which is 200 to 3,000 times the values quoted in Table 33. Part of this ratio is explicable simply by the slower motion of the large molecules. The molecular weight of the rapidly penetrating molecules is ≤ 300, that of the polymers 10,000 to 150,000.

The fluxes of macromolecules are orders of magnitude smaller than for small molecules. Since hair and duct shunt pathways are important for transport of macromolecules, rabbit skin, with its large area fraction of hair follicles, may be a poor model for human skin.

T. Compound Group Comparisons

The previous sections have dealt with individual or small groups of compounds. However,

Table 33
PERMEABILITY OF SKIN TO
POLYMERS, CALCULATED FROM
THEIR PENETRATION OF EXCISED
SKIN[153]

Molecule	Contact time (hr)	Permeability constant (ncm/min)
Rabbit skin		
Human serum albumin	24	63 ± 7 (8)
Human serum albumin (in situ)	6	23 ± 5 (5)
Polyvinyl pyrrolidone	6	6 ± 2 (5)
Dextran fraction 10	24	108 ± 53 (6)
Dextran fraction 150	24	40 ± 17 (6)
Human skin		
Human serum albumin	24	24 ± 2 (4)
Polyvinyl pyrrolidone	6	3 (1)

Note: The mean of each set of observations and its standard
error are given, with the number of experiments in
parentheses.

Table 34
IN VITRO PERMEATION OF RAT SKIN
FROM PETROLATUM VEHICLE[12]

Test compound	Permeability constant (cm/hr)	Percentage of applied dose
Urea	1.6×10^{-5} (1)	7.2 (1)
Acetylsalicylic acid	6.5×10^{-4} (4.1)	29.0 (4.0)
Benzoic acid	3.5×10^{-4} (21.9)	49.1 (6.8)

Note: Values of the $\bar{x}$ of four or five determinations. The relative
permeability of the compounds with each method of cal-
culation is given in parentheses.

many investigations deal with large numbers of materials. Since the results are expressed
differently, the tabulations are presented as separate entities.

1. Benzoic Acid, Acetylsalicylic Acid, Urea, and Caffeine

Bronaugh et al.[12,155] studied the percutaneous absorption of benzoic acid, acetylsalicylic
acid, urea, and caffeine through rat skin after application in a petrolatum vehicle. For
comparative purposes, they selected compounds that had previously been examined in permeability studies by other investigators.[11,112] Absorption was measured in vivo from urinary
excretion data and in vitro with excised skin in diffusion cells over a 5-day period. A
comparison of their data, calculated in terms of permeability constants and percentages of
the applied dose, is shown in Table 34.

The in vivo rate determination and a comparison of the in vivo and in vitro k_p values for
caffeine and ASA are shown in Table 35. Since similar values were obtained in vivo,
permeability measurements of these compounds with excised skin appear reliable.

A comparison of the data with those from other studies with human skin is shown in

Table 35
IN VIVO VS. IN VITRO PERCUTANEOUS ABSORPTION
THROUGH RAT SKIN[a][12]

Test compound	Rate (ng/hr/cm²) Body	Rate (ng/hr/cm²) Urine	Permeability constant (cm/hr) In vivo	Permeability constant (cm/hr) In vitro
Caffeine	16.3	27.8	2.1×10^{-4} (7)	3.1×10^{-4} (6)
Acetylsalicylic acid	0	11.4	5.2×10^{-5} (7)	6.5×10^{-5} (5)

[a] Compounds in a petrolatum vehicle were applied to a 2.0-cm² area of skin on the living animals and in diffusion cells. Results are the means of the number of determinations in parentheses.

Table 36
COMPARISON OF PERMEATION VALUES WITH THOSE OF
OTHER STUDIES

Test compound	Percentage of applied dose In vivo Rat (petrolatum)	In vivo Human[a] (acetone)	In vitro Rat (petrolatum)	In vitro Human[b] (acetone)
Benzoic acid	37.1	42.6	49.1	44.9
Acetylsalicylic acid	24.8	21.8	29.0	40.5
Urea	8.1	6.0	7.2	11.1

[a] Values from Feldmann and Maibach.[112]
[b] Values from Franz.[11]

Table 36. The results appear to be similar in spite of some major differences in the studies. Differences in type of skin and vehicle are indicated in the table and, in addition, there were differences in the duration of contact of the applied compounds with the skin.

2. Griseofulvin and Proquazone

Franz et al.[156] studied the in vivo percutaneous absorption of the antifungal agent, griseofulvin, and the antiinflammatory agent, proquazone in rats. The ability of glycerinformal, a nonvolatile and well-tolerated solvent, to dissolve griseofluvin as well as proquazone in reasonable amounts, together with the observations that monoglycerides of medium chain length promote the percutaneous absorption of drugs prompted the Franz group to investigate the transdermal absorption of griseofulvin and of proquazone from ointments containing glycerinformal together with monoglycerides. The ointments were applied topically on the back of bile cannulated rats. The total amount absorbed percutaneously and the permeability constants of both drugs were considerably higher for the ointments than for simple solutions of the drugs without monoglycerides. As presented in Table 37, the total amount of radioactivity excreted with the bile and the urine after dorsal administration of the ointments in cannulated rats is about 18 times higher for griseofulvin and about six times higher for proquazone than after administration of the corresponding solutions. This is despite the higher initial concentrations in the latter. The remarkable enhancement of the percutaneous absorption of both drugs by the ointment formulations is also reflected by the permeability constants Kp, calculated from the steady state flux in the bile (Table 37). The total amount of radioactivity penetrated into the epidermis and the deeper layers of isolated human skin

Table 37

**EXCRETION OF RADIOACTIVITY WITH THE BILE AND THE URINE (0-72 hr)
AFTER DORSAL ADMINISTRATION IN CANNULATED RATS[156]**

Dosage form	Bile ($\bar{x} \pm$ S.E.M.)	Urine ($\bar{x} \pm$ S.E.M.)	Total ($\bar{x} \pm$ S.E.M.)	n[b]	Permeability constant[a] Kp (cm/hr)
	Amount excreted in % of dose				
[3]H-Griseofulvin					
Solution	2.5 ± 0.3	0.7 ± 0.3	3.2 ± 0.2	5	$3.64 \pm 0.57 \times 10^{-5}$
Ointment	42.8 ± 3.0	11.8 ± 2.0	54.6 ± 4.0	6	$2.00 \pm 0.16 \times 10^{-3}$
[3]H-Proquazone					
Solution	5.2 ± 0.2	2.1 ± 0.4	7.3 ± 0.3	5	$3.57 \pm 0.24 \times 10^{-4}$
Ointment	30.8 ± 1.7	12.4 ± 1.4	43.2 ± 1.3	13	$1.03 \pm 0.06 \times 10^{-3}$

[a]   Minimum value calculated from the steady state flux with the bile.
[b]   Number of experiments

from the same ointment composition represents only about 10% for griseofulvin and only about 2% for proquazone. The medium flow rate through isolated human skin is about six times higher for proquazone than for griseofulvin due to the higher initial concentration of the former.

3. Miscellaneous

Pioneering work was done by Feldman and Maibach[112] who studied the percutaneous penetration of 21 organic chemicals. The experimental method consisted of the application of the chemical to the human forearm and quantitating its penetration through the skin by its appearance in urine. Table 38 gives the recovery rate data after topical administration for each time period and the number of subjects, total recovery (in percent of the applied dose) and standard deviation.

Figure 9 gives the total 5-day absorption expressed as percent of the applied dose. These are listed in order of magnitude. There was a great diversity in the ability of the chemicals to penetrate human skin. Absorption of greater than 40% was noted with DNCB, caffeine, and benzoic acid. Nicotinic acid, hippuric acid, and thiourea penetrated in a quantity less than 1% of the applied dose. Closely related compounds showed great differences in penetration. Benzoic acid was absorbed at 200 times the amount of its glycine conjugate — hippuric acid. Nicotinic acid barely penetrated; 10% of its amide, nicotinamide, penetrated. This suggests that molecules may be tailored to decrease or increase penetration as needed for the most suitable biological function; no chemical shows complete absorption. Presumably, the balance is lost from the epidermal surface. With most compounds the surface loss rate must exceed the absorption rate, for the latter are generally below 50%.

Succeeding authors sought to corroborate the Feldman data. Franz[11] repeated the work using excised human skin. Table 39 compares the results. Several things are immediately evident from the data presented in the table. Quantitative agreement between the two methods is far from perfect. This is particularly true with compounds of low permeability; numbers 1 through 3 in the table, where the in vitro nicotinic acid figure differs by an order of magnitude from its in vivo counterpart. Compounds of high permeability are in much better agreement, and six compounds differ by less than a factor of two. Caffeine and nicotinamide are the only members of this group for which the agreement is not good. Although the absence of exact quantitative agreement between the two methods is evident, a trend toward positive correlation can be noted.

This work demonstrates that the study of percutaneous absorption in excised human skin indeed gives information which is relevant to its living counterpart. When equivalent tech-

Table 38
ABSORPTION AFTER TOPICAL ADMINISTRATION[112]

Steroid	Absorption rate (% dose/hr) Time (hr)						Total absorption		
	0-12	12-14	24-48	48-72	72-96	96-120	% of dose	SD	% of subjects
Acetylsalicylic acid	0.141	0.438	0.334	0.147	0.076	0.060	21.81	3.11	3
Benzoic acid	3.036	0.340	0.055	0.000	0.000	0.000	42.62	16.45	6
Butter yellow	0.215	0.685	0.289	0.083	0.054	0.022	21.57	4.88	4
Caffeine	0.559	1.384	0.855	0.109	0.032	0.014	47.56	20.99	12
Chloramphenicol	0.007	0.019	0.021	0.022	0.015	0.012	2.04	2.46	6
Colchicine	0.036	0.038	0.033	0.040	0.025	0.004	3.69	2.50	6
Dinitrochlorobenzene	3.450	0.565	0.134	0.045	0.018	0.009	53.14	12.41	4
Diethyltoluamide	0.773	0.331	0.084	0.036	0.016	0.012	16.71	5.10	4
Hexachlorophene	0.029	0.031	0.020	0.028	0.034	0.030	3.10	1.09	7
Hippuric acid	0.005	0.003	0.001	0.001	0.001	0.001	0.21	0.09	7
Malathion	0.313	0.170	0.044	0.017	0.011	0.006	7.84	2.71	7
Methylcholanthrene	0.062	0.329	0.258	0.127	0.064	0.045	16.81	5.16	3
Nicotinic acid	0.000	0.002	0.001	0.001	0.002	0.007	0.34	0.09	3
Nicotinamide	0.019	0.168	0.177	0.088	0.052	0.031	11.08	6.17	7
Nitrobenzene	0.022	0.022	0.013	0.013	0.011	0.006	1.53	0.84	6
Paraaminobenzoic acid	0.159	0.648	0.444	0.196	0.058	0.044	28.37	2.43	13
Phenol	0.254	0.091	0.010	0.601	0.000	0.000	4.40	2.43	3
Potassium thiocyanate	0.051	0.060	0.078	0.097	0.100	0.093	10.15	6.60	6
Salicylic acid	0.116	0.535	0.356	0.156	0.080	0.033	22.78	13.25	17
Thiourea	0.046	0.035	0.010	0.008	0.007	0.007	0.88	0.22	3
Urea	0.008	0.021	0.051	0.073	0.075	0.034	5.99	1.91	4

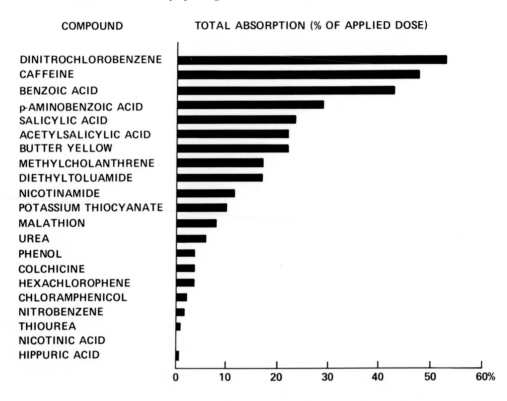

FIGURE 9.   The total absorption of the applied dose. The forearm was the test site. These data represent the amount of isotope present in urine in 5 days after cutaneous application. The applied dose was 4 μg/cm². [112]

Table 39
TOTAL ABSORPTION (EXPRESSED AS % OF APPLIED DOSE) [11]

Compound	In vivo[a]	In vitro[b]
Hippuric acid	0.2 ± 0.1 [7]	1.2 (0.8, 2.7) [15]
Nicotinic acid	0.3 ± 0.1 [3]	3.3 (0.7, 8.3) [19]
Thiourea	0.9 ± 0.2 [3]	3.4 (2.4, 5.5) [52]
Chloramphenicol	2.0 ± 2.5 [6]	2.9 (1.0, 5.7) [12]
Phenol	4.4 ± 2.4 [3]	10.9 (7.7, 26) [7]
Urea	6.0 ± 1.9 [4]	11.1 (5.2, 29) [22]
Nicotinamide	11.1 ± 6.2 [7]	28.8 (16, 65) [21]
Acetylsalicylic acid	21.8 ± 3.1 [3]	40.5 (17, 49)[14]
Salicylic acid	22.8 ± 13.2 [17]	12.0 (2.3, 23) [10]
Benzoic acid	42.6 ± 21.0 [12]	44.9 (29, 53) [18]
Caffeine	47.6 ± 21.0 [12]	9.0 (5.5, 20)[17]
Dinitrochlorobenzene	53.1 ± 12.4 [4]	27.5 (19, 33) [18]

[a]   Mean = SD. The figure in brackets is the number of subjects studied.
[b]   Median with 95% confidence interval given in parentheses.

niques are used, the data obtained from the in vitro preparations of skin correlate well with those obtained in vivo. Specifically, the data presented demonstrate that the in vitro technique is capable of differentiating compounds of low permeability from those of high permeability and ranking them in an order which closely approximates that seen in vivo. Moreover, there is excellent correlation between the kinetics of the absorption process as determined in vitro and in vivo, and therein lies a strong argument to support the validity of the in vitro method.

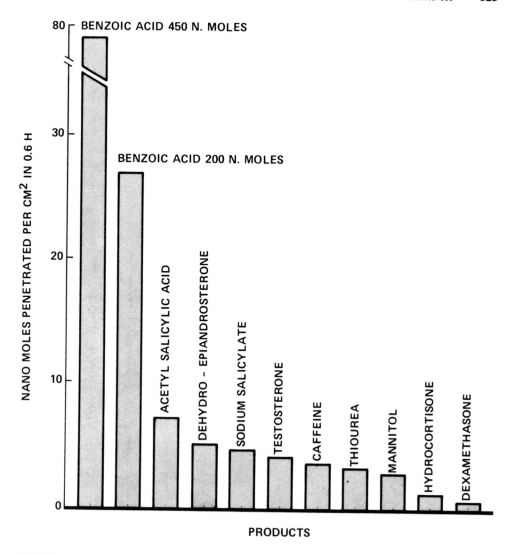

FIGURE 10. Total percutaneous absorption levels (nmol/cm²) of the products tested 96 hr after their topical application on the hairless rat.[157]

What is currently lacking is information which speaks to the quantitative correlation between in vitro and in vivo absorption. Although the data presented demonstrate an unmistakable trend toward quantitative agreement, when considering all the data, they do not answer the question conclusively.

Rougier[157] investigated a similar group of chemicals, in vivo in the hairless rat. The percutaneous absorption results, in agreement with those obtained in the literature, show that after 96 hr there are large differences in the amounts of substances that have penetrated through the skin (Figure 10). The rank order established in humans by Feldman et al.[158] in the level of steroid penetration — dexamethasone, hydrocortisone, testosterone, and dehydroepiandrosterone — is seen in results in the rat. Furthermore, hydrocortisone penetrates five times less than testosterone and dehydroepiandrosterone which have almost identical penetrating properties. There is also agreement with previous data for acetylsalicylic acid and benzoic acid, the latter known to be very well absorbed.[112] Likewise, it is known that acetylsalicylic acid and salicylic acid have similar penetrating properties,[112] whereas their sodium salts exhibit diminished penetration.[159] Bartek et al.[9] compared percutaneous ab-

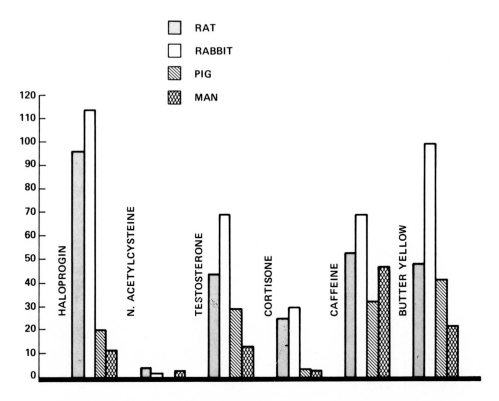

FIGURE 11.   Percutaneous absorption of several compounds in rat, rabbit, pig, and man.[53]

sorption in rats, rabbits, miniature swine, and man (Figure 11). Haloprogin (3-iodo-2-propynl-2,4,5-trichlorophenyl ether), a topical antifungal agent, was completely absorbed by the rat. Penetration through the skin of pigs and humans was minimal in all species. Cortisone, a minimal penetrant through the skin of man and miniature swine, was well absorbed by the rat and rabbit. Caffeine readily penetrated the skin of all species. With Butter Yellow, penetration through rabbit skin was much greater than through skin of the other three species. Testosterone penetration was greatest in the rabbit, followed by the rat and then the pig, which was closest to man. This study showed rabbit skin to be the most permeable to topically applied compounds, followed closely by rat skin. In contrast, it appears that the permeability of the skin of the miniature swine is closer to that of human skin. Clearly, percutaneous absorption in the rabbit and rat would not be predictive of that in man. It is not known whether the subtle differences seen between pig and human skin were due to methodology (site of application, shaving) or to the skin itself. However, generally the pig appears to be a good predictor of percutaneous absorption in man.

Bronaugh[155] tabulated the results of a number of investigators which compare the permeability of the compounds in human and animal skin. The permeability is expressed relative to the absorption found with human skin in each study (Table 40).

All these studies show that values for even the most permeable skin, such as rabbit or mouse, are often well within an order of magnitude of values for human skin. The fact that butter yellow permeates pig skin only 1.9 times faster than it does human skin is not as significant when it is considered that rat and rabbit skins are only 2.2 and 4.6 times more permeable, respectively. In addition, the permeability of benzoic acid in hairless mouse skin was only twice that of human skin, and this result was also obtained with the skin of the Swiss mouse. It thus appears that, depending on the compound of interest and the vehicle used, values that are not too dissimilar from those with human skin might be obtained with the skin of a number of animal species.

Table 40
PERMEABILITY OF ANIMAL SKIN RELATIVE TO HUMAN SKIN[a,b][155]

Reference and compound	Pig	Monkey	Rat	Guinea pig	Hairless mouse	Mouse	Rabbit
Bartek et al.[9]							
n-Acetylcysteine	2.5		1.4				0.8
Benzoic acid[c]		1.4					
Butter yellow	1.9		2.2				4.6
Caffeine	0.7		1.1				1.5
Cortisone	1.2		7.3				9.0
Haloprogin	2.6		3.7				4.4
Hydrocortisone[c]		1.6					
Testosterone[c]	2.2	1.4	3.6				5.3
Tregear[160]							
Ethylenebromide	0.8		2.3	1.5			
Paraoxon	1.4		3.3	3.0			
Thioglycolic acid	3.3		3.0	2.3			
Water	1.4			1.0			3.3
Andersen et al.[161]							
Benzoic acid				0.7			
Hydrocortisone				1.3			
Testosterone				2.6			
Chowhan and Pritchard[143]							
Naproxin			2.3				3.5
Durrheim et al.[43]							
Butanol					1.8		
Ethanol					1.5		
Octanol					0.6		
Stoughton[162]							
Betamethasone					1.3		
5-Fluorouracil					1.1		
Hydrocortisone					1.5		
Data from present study[155]							
Acetylsalicylic acid	1.2		1.0		4.9	8.7	
Benzoic acid	0.2		0.6		2.0	2.0	
Urea	1.5		4.8		0.9	5.8	

[a] Values from human skin in all studies were assigned a value of 10.
[b] Values from Bartek et al.[9] and Andersen et al.[161] were obtained in vivo. Other results are from experiments using excised skin.
[c] Data taken completely or in part from Wester and Maibach.[163]

Bronaugh[68] collected the permeability constants of cosmetic ingredients through excised human skin (Table 41). Scala et al.[131] compiled a variety of data on a wide series of compounds (Table 42).

Higuchi[29] used a thermodynamic approach to relate molecular structure and rate of percutaneous absorption. He notes that the maximum rate of delivery through the skin is closely limited to that resulting from the thermodynamic activity of the pure drug substance. A number of different chemical substances and the approximate thermodynamic activities of their pure states are listed in Table 43. If all other factors are equal, the maximal expected rate of percutaneous delivery achievable will be proportional to the values such as given in the table. On this basis, norethindrone acetate, for example, can be expected to be delivered approximately 40 times faster than norethindrone alcohol and chloroform roughly 100 times that of ethanol.

Table 41
PERMEABILITY CONSTANTS OF COSMETIC INGREDIENTS WITH EXCISED HUMAN SKIN[68]

Compound	KP (cm/hr × 10^5)	Type of vehicle	Ref.
Benzoic acid	87	Petrolatum	155
Caffeine	80	Petrolatum	155
Chlorocresol	5496	Aqueous	92
Chloroxylenol	5404	Aqueous	92
Estradiol	30	Aqueous	96
	520	Aqueous	69
	389	Aqueous	167
Ethanol	100	Aqueous	33
Hexanol	1300	Aqueous	33
Methylhydroxybenzoate	912	Aqueous	92
β-Naphthol	2790	Aqueous	92
2-Nitro-*p*-phenylenediamine	50	Aqueous	165
Phenol	822	Aqueous	92
Propanol	140	Aqueous	33
Resorcinol	24	Aqueous	92
p-Phenylenediamine	24	Aqueous	166
o-Phenylenediamine	45	Aqueous	166
Testosterone	40	Aqueous	96
Thymol	5280	Aqueous	92
Urea	0.3	Petrolatum	92
Water	100	Aqueous	33
	159	Aqueous	164

III. DRUG CLASSES AND PERMEATION

A. Anesthetics

It is apparent from several studies in humans that the intact skin acts as a barrier to the easy penetration of topically applied local anesthetics.[171-173]

1. Lidocaine

Akerman et al.[174] studied the capacity of lidocaine to affect local anesthesia of the intact skin of the guinea pig. The results show that epicutaneously applied lidocaine could overcome the skin barrier to penetration and reach deeper layers containing nerve fibers in order to exert a true local anesthetic action. The degree of percutaneous local anesthesia increased as the concentration of lidocaine in the applied solution or the time of application was increased. Lidocaine was taken up to a greater extent and was more effective when used as the base in an alcoholic mixture than as the salt in water at equal concentrations. This probably reflects the character of the stratum corneum as a lipid composite membrane, through which lipid-soluble substances may pass more easily than lipid-insoluble substances, especially electrolytes. The fact that use of compounds such as dimethylacetamide and dimethylformamide as solvents for lidocaine resulted in increased skin penetration and higher efficacy is in agreement with the observations that these dipolar aprotic solvents are known to facilitate penetration of the skin barrier by steroids and griseofulvin.[175,176]

Pretreatment with dimethylacetamide resulted in a more intense anesthetic effect than that following pretreatment with an alcoholic solvent mixture, which suggests that the penetration of lidocaine was enhanced by these solvents by different mechanisms. Dipolar aprotic solvents differ from water or alcohol in that they have a tendency to accept rather than donate protons. They can thus compete effectively for hydrogen donor molecules, even with water. Thus, it seems reasonable to suppose that dipolar aprotic solvents may interact strongly

Table 42
PERMEABILITY OF THE SKIN[131]

Material	Conc	pH	Type of skin	Duration of diffusion	Permeability constant (cm/min × 10^{-6})	Ref.
Water	—	—	Rabbit	—	147	3
Na laurate	5 mM	7.5	Human	12—23 hr	10	138
		8.0			3.8	
		9.0			1.0	
		10.0			1.0	
		11.0			1.0	
		12.0			7.5	
K palmitate	40 mM	9—10	Human	7 days	0.3	140
K oleate					5.0	
K laurate					20.0	
K octanoate					10.0	
Thioglycollic acid	560 mM	—	Rabbit	—	110.0	3
	5.6 M				850.0	
Na$^+$, K$^+$, Br$^-$	155 mM	7.0	Human	5—8 hr	0.6—1.0	167
PO$_4$			Pig		3.0—30.0	
			Rabbit		20.0—60.0	
Hg^{++}	40—80 mM	—	Guinea pig	5 hr	14.0—45.0	168
CrO$_4^{++}$	0.5 mM—4.9 M	7—8.5	Guinea pig	5 hr	20.0—30.0	169
Methanol	2.5 mM—12.4 M	—	Rabbit	1—2 hr	42.0	126
			Rabbit dermis		1960.0	
Ethanol	10—50 mM	—	Rabbit		44.0	170
			Rabbit dermis		1410.0	
Butanol	100-200 mM	—	Human	4—5 hr	42.0	
Pentanol	100-200 mM	—	Human		100.0	
Thiourea	10-50 mM	—	Rabbit	1—2 hr	2.9	126
			Rabbit dermis		1110.0	
Glycerol	10-50 mM	—	Rabbit	1—2 hr	3.9	
			Rabbit dermis		910.0	
Urea	10-50 mM	—	Rabbit	1—2 hr	2.4	
			Rabbit dermis		1200.0	

Table 42 (continued)
PERMEABILITY OF THE SKIN[131]

Material	Conc	pH	Type of skin	Duration of diffusion	Permeability constant (cm/min × 10⁻⁶)	Ref.
Glucose	10-50 mM	—	Rabbit	1—2 hr	0.9	
			Rabbit dermis		700.0	
Ethyl iodide	10-50 mM	—	Rabbit	1—2 hr	91.0	3
Ethylene bromide	5.0 mM	—	Rabbit	—	5.8	
	100%	—	Rabbit	—	4.4	
Tri-ethyl phosphate	3—30 mM	—	Rabbit	—	26.0	
	100%	—	Rabbit	—	1.9	
Tri-n-propyl phosphate	100%	—	Human	18—20 hr	0.8	5
Tri-n-butyl phosphate	100%	—	Rabbit	18—20 hr	2.1	3
			Human		0.2	5

Table 43
APPROXIMATE THERMODYNAMIC
ACTIVITIES OF SOME TYPICAL
PURE ORGANIC COMPOUNDS[29]

Substances	Activity of (mol/ℓ) Pure State
Acetanilide	0.0009
Benzene	11.2
1-Butanol	0.20
Carbazole	0.0015
Chloroform	12.4
Ethanol	0.135
Ethyl ether	9.55
1-Hexanol	0.41
Hydrocortisone	$<2 \times 10^{-6}$
Hydrocortisone acetate	$<2 \times 10^{-6}$
4-Iodophenol	0.0156
Methanol	0.1
Methyl testosterone	0.00123
4-Nitrophenol	0.00036
Norethindrone	0.000071
Norethindrone acetate	0.00275
Phenol	0.67
Phthalic anhydride	0.00050
Picric acid	0.00030
2,4,6-Triiodophenol	0.0050

with the stratum corneum, especially the proteins, and this may cause a looser structure resulting in an increased permeability of the stratum corneum.[38,177]

Tertiary aliphatic amides unsubstituted in the *N*-alkyl groups were all effective vehicles for lidocaine, though dimethylacetamide and dimethylformamide appeared to be best in this respect. Amides with a high electron density at the amide carbonyl should be effective proton acceptors. However, introduction of ether or ester functions into one of the *N*-alkyl groups, or its replacement by an alkoxyl group, such as is the case with the derivatives of dimethylacetamide substituted in the dimethylamine moiety, can result in a withdrawal of electron density from the amide carbonyl with a resulting decrease in the capacity of this group to accept protons and interact with the stratum corneum proteins. This may explain the poor vehicle effect of these substituted amides. A similar argument may be used to explain the inferiority of morpholones compared to the pyrrolidones and also absence of effect with *N*-acetylmorpholine. Of course, it must be remembered that other physicochemical factors such as steric and conformational effects, molecular weight and lipid solubility may also be operative.

Secondary amides such as *N*-methylacetamide exist in the transconformation and intermolecular hydrogen bonding can result in an extended structure (a loose polymer) which would not interact as effectively as dipolar solvents with proteins and, due to the large effective molecular size, would have retarded penetration properties. This may explain why *N*-methylacetamide was ineffective as a penetration enhancer for lidocaine. However, 2-pyrrolidone, which also contains a labile proton was a surprisingly effective vehicle. In this cyclic molecule, the amide bond has the cis conformation, and hydrogen bonding with another lactam molecule gives a dimeric structure. Thus, although intermolecular hydrogen bonding will prevent as effective competition for protein hydrogen bonding as with dipolar aprotic solvents, the relatively small effective molecular size may allow reasonably facile penetration of the skin. This investigation[174] suggests that aliphatic amides unsubstituted in

Table 44
EFFECT OF POLYOXYETHYLENE NONYLPHENOLS ON BENZOCAINE PENETRATION THROUGH HAIRLESS MOUSE SKIN[150]

Polyoxyethylene chain length (n)	Surfactant conc		Total benzocaine conc (mg/mℓ)	Average flux mg/hr·cm^2 × 10^5 ±SD
	% w/v	M		
—	—	—	1.262	60.0 ± 3.9
9	1.4	0.0227	—	59.1 ± 3.2
15	0.2	0.00227	1.265	51.8 ± 3.2
15	1.0	0.01135	2.168	67.5 ± 8.3
15	2.0	0.0277	3.308	58.7 ± 3.5
30	3.5	0.0227	—	63.6 ± 1.0
50	5.5	0.0227	4.275	58.5 ± 7.0

Table 45
SKIN PENETRATION OF BENZOCAINE FROM AQUEOUS SUSPENSIONS[151]

Formulation	Benzocaine conc (% w/v)	Gelling agent (% w/v)		Surfactant conc (M × 10^3)		Flux ± SD, mg/hr/cm^2 × 10^3
		Hydroxypropyl cellulose	Xanthan gum	n = 50	n = 15	
A	1	2	—	—	22.7	97.3 ± 6.5
B	5	2	—	—	22.7	109.8 ± 4.3
C	10	2	—	—	22.7	98.6 ± 8.1
D	1	—	0.4	—	22.7	88.9 ± 7.3
E	5	—	0.4	—	22.7	97.3 ± 8.7
F	5	—	0.4	22.7	—	108.6 ± 6.3
G	5	—	0.4	—	22.7	107.8 ± 6.2

the *N*-alkyl groups, e.g., dimethylacetamide, with a strong tendency to accept protons improve the percutaneous penetration of lidocaine. Substitution in the *N*-alkyl groups of such amides results in a marketed deterioration of this property and cyclic amides are less effective.

2. Benzocaine

Dalvi and Zatz[150] studied the penetration of benzocaine (ethylaminobenzoate) through hairless mouse skin in the presence of nonionic surface active agents (polyoxyethylene nonylphenols — Table 44). Benzocaine flux from saturated solutions was not affected by differences in either polyoxyethylene chain length or surfactant concentration. It was concluded that wetting and skin-surfactant interaction do not play a role in modulating benzocaine penetration through hairless mouse skin. If either effect had been operative, the penetration flux from solutions containing surfactant would have been higher than from a simple aqueous solution. All of the experimental data can be reconciled by consideration of the free benzocaine concentration. The saturated solutions contain the same concentration of free benzocaine and exhibit the same penetration flux. In the solution systems studied, benzocaine penetration was directly related to free benzocaine concentration and not to the total benzocaine concentration.

The same authors[151] extended their studies of benzocaine penetration through hairless mouse skin to aqueous gel suspensions to determine the rate-limiting step in penetration and the influence of nonionic surfactants in these systems. Details of the suspension formulations are listed in Table 45. The flux values showed that drug concentration, gelling agent, and

Table 46
DATA FOR INDOMETHACIN[182]

Indomethacin 1% form (base)	Carrageenin paw edema		UV-erythema		
	Efficacy	Serum levels $\mu g/m\ell$	Efficacy	Serum levels $\mu g/m\ell$	Skin levels $\mu g/g$
Ointment (lipophilic)	+ +	0.14 ± 0.1	+ +	0.07	0.39 ± 0.07
Cream (O/W emulsion)	+ +	0.18 ± 0.01	+ +	0.08	0.68 ± 0.08^a
Gel (carboxyvinylpolymer)	+ + +[b]	0.32 ± 0.02^c	+ + +[b]	0.11	0.94 ± 0.18^d

[a] $p < 0.01$ vs. ointment.
[b] $p < 0.05$ vs. ointment.
[c] $p < 0.01$ vs. ointment, $p < 0.05$ vs. cream.
[d] $p < 0.01$ vs. ointment and cream.

surfactant concentration had no statistically significant effect on flux. No influence of the surfactants on skin membrane integrity was evident. These results are similar to those with saturated benzocaine solutions.[150] However, there is a surprising difference in the magnitude of the penetration values when saturated solutions are compared to suspensions. Mean benzocaine flux from saturated solution was ~ 60 $\mu g/hr/cm^2$ whereas the average flux for suspensions was 101 $\mu g/hr/cm^2$. This difference was unexpected since the free benzocaine concentration which provides the driving force for diffusion should have been the same in both types of preparation.

B. Nonsteroidal Anti-inflammatory Agents (NSAID)

Nonsteroidal anti-inflammatory agents (NSAID) are widely used for the treatment of various inflammatory diseases. Oral administration is often accompanied by a variety of side effects. Efforts have been made to avoid these by topical administration.

1. Indomethacin

Some NSAIDS are known to distribute preferentially to the inflamed tissue.[178] Tissue levels of indomethacin (ID) in the deep muscle layer after topical application are close to those in the synovial fluid from arthritic patients after an oral dose of 50 mg.[179] The presence of indomethacin in the muscle and the skin of guinea pigs was demonstrated through percutaneous absorption from an ointment.[180]

Two studies[181,182] focused on the comparative percutaneous absorption of ID from varied vehicles. Shima et al.[182] studied permeation from a gel and varied ointments. The concentration of ID absorbed from the gel ointment was the highest, that is, 38.5 $\mu g/g$ skin and 1.1 $\mu g/g$ muscle. On the other hand, the extent of absorption of ID from other ointments decreased in the following order: absorptive ointment = hydrophilic ointment > white petrolatum ointment = plastibase ointment > macrogel ointment. Kyuki[181] noted that when ID in ointment cream and gel bases is percutaneously applied to carrageenin-injected or UV-radiated sites, its anti-inflammatory actions in both models are stronger in gel than in ointment. ID gel produces significantly higher serum levels in the carrageenin model and higher skin levels in the UV-erythema model than indomethacin ointment (Table 46).

2. Flufenamic Acid

Percutaneous absorption of flufenamic acid and the resulting anti-inflammatory activity has been shown using animal and human models.[183-185] Hwang and Danti[186] studied the effect of surfactants on the permeation. Eight nonionic surface-active agents were incorporated at a concentration of 10% into a white petrolatum ointment base containing 10%

Table 47
AUC$_{0-8}$ FOR PLASMA CONCENTRATION(S) OF
FLUFENAMIC ACID VS. TIME FOR
FORMULATIONS WITH AND WITHOUT DMSO[a] [186]

Surfactant	I[b]	II[c]
None	7.400 ± 1.332	21.784 ± 4.369
Sorbitan monopalmitate	5.421 ± 0.730	38.721 ± 1.016
Sorbitan trioleate	38.511 ± 12.976	123.194 ± 1.096
Polyoxyl 8 stearate	16.532 ± 4.131	64.462 ± 3.662
Polyoxyl 40 stearate	7.456 ± 0.373	11.751 ± 0.254
Polyoxyethylene 20 cetyl ether	1.789 ± 0.266	37.753 ± 5.044
Polyoxyethylene 2 oleyl ether	23.066 ± 8.460	109.314 ± 19.114
Poloxamer 184	2.610 ± 0.610	10.023 ± 0.608
Poloxamer 231	8.455 ± 2.749	26.384 ± 6.538

[a]   Percutaneous absorption in rabbits; average of three determinations.
[b]   Flufenamic acid, surfactant, and white petrolatum.
[c]   Flufenamic acid, surfactant, dimethyl sulfoxide, and white petrolatum.

flufenamic acid with or without DMSO. Percutaneous absorption was studied by determining the plasma concentration of flufenamic acid in rabbits at regular intervals for 8 hr following application of the ointment. The absorption was significantly increased when sorbitan trioleate, polyoxyl-8-stearate, or polyoxyethylene-2-oleyl-ether were added to the ointment containing flufenamic acid and white petrolatum. The percutaneous absorption was also increased significantly when sorbitan monopalmitate, sorbitan trioleate, polyoxyl-8-stearate, polyoxyethylene-20-cetyl ether, or polyoxyethylene-2-oleyl-ether were added to the ointment containing DMSO, flufenamic acid and white petrolatum (Table 47).

3. Parfenac

Schaefer and Stuettgen[187] studied the percutaneous absorption of Parfenac, *p*-butoxphenylacetohydroxamic acid, into human skin. The drug was absorbed rapidly in vitro and in vivo from both a cream and ointment. The flow rate for the 5% formulation through the horny layer in vitro was higher for the ointments (3.8×10^{-8} mol/cm^2/hr) than from the cream (7×10^{-9} mol/cm^2/hr).

Schiantarelli et al.[188] used pharmacological end points to determine the topical and the percutaneous anti-inflammatory potencies of a topical formulation of piroxicam using as reference standards nonsteroidal and steroidal anti-inflammatory drugs having the same exicipient base (indomethacin and hydrocortisone acetate) or as topical formulations (ketoprofen and oxyphenbutazone). As shown in Table 48, the application of the topical formulation containing 5% piroxicam induced a slight (17.3%) but significant inhibition of croton oil edema whereas the 1% piroxicam preparation and the 5 and 1% indomethacin formulations induced no significant antiedemal effect. The topical application of 1% hydrocortisone acetate induced intense (71%) antiedemal activity, in line with previous findings, i.e., that the croton oil test is the method of choice when testing nonsteroid anti-inflammatory drugs (NSAID) for cutaneous anti-inflammatory potency.[189,190]

4. Naproxen

Chowhan et al.[143,152] evaluated the effect of surfactants on percutaneous absorption of naproxen through excised human skin using a simple aqueous gel system. The results of

Table 48
CROTON OIL EAR TEST IN THE MOUSE. EFFECTS OF PIROXICAM, INDOMETHACIN, AND HYDROCORTISONE ACETATE TOPICALLY APPLIED MIXED WITH CROTON OIL[188]

Active principle of topical formulation	Conc of active principle (%)	Quantity of active principle applied (mg)	No. of animals	% Inhibition of edema	p
Piroxicam	1	0.09	25	3.3	NS
Piroxicam	5	0.44	52	17.3	<0.05
Indometacin	1	0.09	20	−2.5	NS
	5	0.44	40	12.7	NS
Hydrocortisone acetate	1	0.09	15	71.0	<0.01

Note: Edema is represented by the difference in weight between the disks taken from the right (treated) ear and the left (untreated) ear. The percent difference between the edema of the treated animals and that of the controls that had received croton oil + excipient only is the edema inhibition.

Table 49
EFFECT OF SURFACTANTS ON NAPROXEN FLUX THROUGH EXCISED HUMAN ABDOMINAL SKIN FROM AQUEOUS GELS[143,152]

Surfactant (conc)	Mean flux (μg/cm^2/hr)	SD	Relative flux
Experiment 1			
No added surfactant (control)	2.82	0.41	1.0
Hexadecylpyridinium chloride (0.5%)	1.26	0.22	0.44
Triethylammonium lauryl sulfate (2%)	2.00	0.81	0.71
Octylphenoxypolyethoxy 5 ethanol (2%)	2.30	0.24	0.82
Dioctyl sodium sulfosuccinate (0.05%)	2.94	0.21	1.04
Experiment 2			
No added surfactant (control)	1.26	0.58	1.0
Sodium lauryl sulfate (4%)	10.45	0.18	8.29
Sodium laurate (4%)	3.17	1.29	2.51
Polysorbate 60 (4%)	1.22	0.11	0.97
Polyoxyethylene 23 lauryl ether (4%)	1.04	0.18	0.83

these experiments are given in Table 49. For comparison, the mean flux of control in each experiment was taken as one and the relative flux was then calculated. The concentration of all surfactants was above the critical micelle concentration (CMC). The effect of nonionic, cationic, and amphoteric surfactants on the relative flux of naproxen was small. The lower relative flux with certain surfactants may be due to the lowering of the thermodynamic activity of naproxen by solubilization of the drug in micelles. The anionic surfactants, sodium laurate and sodium lauryl sulfate, increased the in vitro flux of naproxen appreciably.

The in vitro mean flux of naproxen through excised human, rat, and rabbit skins is given in Table 50. The in vitro mean flux of the control experiments indicates that the excised

Table 50

EFFECT OF SURFACTANTS ON THE IN VITRO FLUX OF NAPROXEN THROUGH EXCISED
HUMAN, RAT, AND RABBIT SKINS FROM AN OIL-IN-WATER CREAM FORMULATION[143]

Surfactant (conc)	Excised human skin			Excised rat skin			Excised rabbit skin		
	Mean flux, $\mu g/cm^2/hr$	SD	Relative flux	Mean flux, $\mu g/cm^2/hr$	SD	Relative flux	Mean flux, $\mu g/cm^2/hr$	SD	Relative flux
No added surfactant (control)	1.66	0.49	1	3.75	0.60	1	5.86	0.55	1
Sodium lauryl sulfate (2%)	5.12	1.86	3.09	4.91	0.79	1.31	10.18	4.78	1.74
Sodium laurate (2%)	7.32	3.69	4.41	6.53	0.18	1.74	20.01	9.00	3.41
Methyldecyl sulfoxide (1%)	17.18	4.32	10.35	5.47	0.54	1.46	24.11	10.34	4.11

human skin was the least permeable and that the excised rabbit skin was most permeable to naproxen. Another important difference in the three types of excised skin was in the lag time. The lag time for the human skin was approximately 100 hr; for the rat and rabbit skins, it was about 14 hr. Although excised rat skin was less permeable than excised rabbit skin, the lag time was similar.

C. Bronchodilator (Cromolyn)

Cromolyn [1,3-*bis*(2-carboxychromon-5-yloxyl)-propan-2-ol, cromoglycic acid] is used primarily in the prophylactic treatment of bronchial asthma. Topically applied sodium cromoglycate was effective in the treatment of atopic eczema in children.[191] However, cromolyn is a highly polar molecule; thus, it has poor bioavailability whether administered orally, parenterally, or by inhalation. Its polar character and short biological half-life make it difficult to have the drug absorbed through and/or concentrate in the skin. Bodor[192] studied the percutaneous absorption of lipophilic prodrugs of cromolyn into the excised skin of the hairless mouse. The prodrugs selected for testing are shown in Table 51. The results of the diffusion studies on these compounds are summarized in Table 52. Although seen in only relatively small amounts (0.5% in 12 hr), cromoglycic acid does penetrate the intact skin significantly. Higher amounts penetrate the skin when the lipoidal prodrugs are used. Thus, the hexanoyloxyethylidene (6), hexanoyloxymethyl (3), and pivalyloxymethyl-nitrate esters (11) all resulted in about 3% of the dose appearing in the receptor phase in the form of cromoglycic acid. It is important to emphasize that the prodrugs did indeed deliver cromoglycic acid; thus, significant metabolism in the skin takes place.

The absorption of cromolyn and some selected prodrugs was confirmed in vivo, using hairless mice. The results are given in Table 53. It is evident that as expected, only negligible amounts are distributed in the various organs and tissues (intestine, bile, fat, etc.). The only significant amounts were found in the skin, urine, and feces, indicating that cromoglycic acid, can indeed, be delivered topically in vivo. As in the case of the diffusion cell studies, the lipoidal-6 resulted in the highest overall delivery (particularly the excreted part), although cromolyn itself showed an apparently better absorption as in vitro.

D. Anticholinergics

1. Hyoscine

Use of anticholinergic drugs in treatment of duodenal ulcers is limited by the side effects of widespread parasympathetic blockade evoked by usual therapeutic doses. A study was conducted into the effectiveness of transdermal delivery of hyoscine methobromide.[193] Nocturnal acid secretions in six patients with healed duodenal ulcers was significantly inhibited. In view of the efficacy of the regimen in inhibiting nocturnal acid secretion (by 75%) and the absence of severe adverse reactions, the investigators suggested that transdermal anticholinergic therapy may represent a valuable alternative for maintenance treatment of duodenal ulcer.

2. Scopolamine

Scopolamine was the first drug administered transdermally. Shaw and Chandrasekaran[194] studied the skin permeation of scopolamine. Table 54 notes that the flux of the free base was greater than the salt. From saturated solutions, permeation of scopolamine base through the dermis was orders of magnitude greater than the rates of permeation through epidermis or whole skin, indicating that the principle resistance to scopolamine permeation resides in the epidermis (Table 54).

E. Antineoplastic Agents

Antineoplastic agents, as a result of their antimitotic potency, have been considered as

Table 51
SELECTED PRODRUGS OF CROMOGLYCIC ACID

Compound	R_1	R_2	R_3	R_4
1	H	O	O	H
2	$-CH_2OCC(CH_3)_3$ (with C=O)	O	O	H
3	$-CH_2OC(CH_2)_4CH_3$ (with C=O)	O	O	H
4	$-CH_2OCCH_2CH_2-$	O	O	H
5	$-CH_2OC(CH_2)_{10}CH_3$ (with C=O)	O	O	H
6	$-CHOC(CH_2)_4CH_3$ (with C=O) $\; | \; CH_3$	O	O	H
7	$-CH_2CN(C_2H_5)_2$ (with C=O)	O	O	H
8	$-CH_2COOC(CH_3)_3$	O	O	H
9	$-CH_2COOH$	O	O	H
10	$-CH(COOC_2H_5)_2$	O	O	H
11	$-CH_2OCC(CH_3)_3$ (with C=O)	O	O	NO_2
12	$-CH_2OC(CH_2)_4CH_3$ (with C=O)	O	O	NO_2
13	$-C_2H_5$	$NOCH_3$	$NOCH_3$	H
14	$-C_2H_5$	$NOCH_3$	O	H
15[a]	$(n-C_4H_9)_3\overset{\oplus}{N}CH_2C_6H_5$	O	O	H

[a] The bis-benzyl-tributylammonium salt of the cromoglycic acid.
From Ref. 192.

Table 52
DIFFUSION OF CROMOGLYCIC ACID (1) AND ITS SELECTED PRODRUGS THROUGH HAIRLESS MOUSE SKIN[a] [192]

Compound cromoglycic acid	Material in the receptor phase[b]		
	Conc (g/mℓ)	g in 40 mℓ	% of dose diffused
1[c]	0.478	19.00	0.50
3	2.629	105.16	2.74
6	2.946	117.83	3.07
7	1.789	71.55	1.86
11	2.761	110.45	2.88
12	1.561	62.44	1.63
13	1.957	78.26	2.04
14	1.978	79.10	2.06
15	1.757	70.27	1.83

[a]   Sample time = 12 hr.
[b]   Only cromoglycic acid 1 was found in the receptor phase, except in the case of 7 and 14 (see text).
[c]   As the disodium salt.

Table 53
IN VIVO DIFFUSION OF TOPICALLY APPLIED CROMOLYN AND ITS SELECTED PRODRUGS[192]

Organ	Compounds (% of dose diffused in 24 hr)			
	7	6	15	1
No. of animals	n = 2	n = 2	n = 1	n = 4
Skin	0.440	0.840	1.950	0.560
Feces	0.660	1.230	0.820	1.105
Urine	0.310	1.450	0.330	0.645
Contents of small intestine	0.008	0.015	0.003	0.028
Contents of large intestine	0.010	0.020	0.007	0.053
Bile	—	—	0.003	—
Blood	—	0.006	0.002	0.014
Small intestine	—	—	—	0.005
Fat	0.050	—	—	—
Muscle	—	0.002	—	—
Carcass	—	0.030	0.141	0.020
Subtotal	1.478	3.593	3.256	2.430
Wash	98.800	103.050	93.820	104.430
Total recovery	100.278	106.643	97.076	106.860

possibly effective agents for hyperkeratotic diseases such as refractory psoriasis. Systemic administration of these compounds is often associated with severe side effects, such as liver toxicity, leukopenia, and bone marrow depression.

1. Hydroxy Urea

Percutaneous administration of hydroxy urea in a 10% cream applied directly to psoriatic lesions has been found to be effective when kept under continuous occlusion for 2 weeks.[195] These results suggested that a topical formulation that would enhance the penetration of hydroxy urea without the need for occlusion might be effective while increasing patient convenience and eliminating systemic toxicities. A cream formulation was developed which

Table 54
SKIN PERMEATION BY SCOPOLAMINE IN SATURATED AQUEOUS SOLUTIONS[194]

Drug form	Skin	Skin thickness (μm)	Steady-state flux (μg/cm²/hr)
Free base	Whole skin	37.5	6.0
	Epidermis	2.0	6.7
	Dermis	35.0	1342
Salt	Whole skin	37.5	0.8
	Dermis	35.0	5710

Table 55
IN VITRO PERCUTANEOUS PENETRATION STUDY — EPIDERMAL MGBG[a] CONTENT[197]

Vehicle	MGBG content of epidermis at 48 hr [μg (mean ± SD)]
Vehicle N	525 ± 81
C_{10}MSO:H_2O (2.5:97.5)	1191 ± 266
Saline	58 ± 25
N-Methylpyrrolidone:isopropyl alcohol:H_2O (43:30:27)	185 ± 85

Note: 10% MGBG in the above vehicles was applied to the epidermal surface of human skin in vitro.

[a]   MGBG = methyl glyoxal *bis*(guanylhydrazone).

contained a DMSO derivative as an absorption enhancer. The formulation markedly accelerated the penetration of hydroxy urea through animal and human skin, in vitro, without occlusion. Shrewsbury et al.[196] followed permeation of the drug through the psoriatic lesions of four patients. Hydroxy urea appeared in both plasma and urine following a 24-hr exposure to the cream. The extent of absorption varied greatly from patient to patient, ranging from 5 to 22% of the dose being absorbed. The rate and extent of absorption appeared to be related to the severity of the disease.

2. Methyl Glyoxal bis(guanylhydrazone)

The antineoplastic agent, methyl glyoxal *bis*(guanylhydrazone) (MGBG) has also been shown to produce partial clinical improvement in psoriasis on topical application. McCullough et al.[197] sought to evaluate the percutaneous penetration of MGBG in vitro on excised human skin.

The percutaneous penetration of 10% MGBG was determined in saline and three other vehicles that have been reported to enhance penetration of various drugs. There was an increase in penetration at 24 and 48 hr in C_{10}MSO and Vehicle N compared to saline (Table 55). Vehicle N produced the maximum rate of MGBG penetration of 3 μg/hr/cm² of skin. There was a dose-dependent increase in MGBG penetration in Vehicle N comparing 0.1, 1 and 10% MGBG penetration at 48 hr. The penetration of 0.1% MGBG in Vehicle N exceeded that of 10% MGBG in saline. Vehicle N and C_{10}MSO vehicles also produced a significant

Table 56
PERCUTANEOUS PENETRATION OF 2%
METHOTREXATE IN HUMAN SKIN IN
VITRO[198]

Vehicle Water	Penetration[a]			
	24 hr		48 hr	
	μg	%	μg	%
Water	6 ± 2	0.05	15 ± 5	0.15
$C_{10}MSO$ (2.5%)	12 ± 10	0.12	36 ± 28	0.36
Vehicle N	50 ± 11	0.50	124 ± 10	1.24

[a] Mean values ± SD for 4 diffusion chambers.

Table 57
COMPARISON OF DIFFUSION OF MTX
THROUGH HAIRLESS MOUSE AND
HUMAN AUTOPSY SKIN IN VITRO
FROM A 0.25% SOLUTION AT pH 8.15[203]

	Flux, J_s (μg/cm²/hr)	Lag time, r
Human autopsy skin	0.034 ± 0.014	11.9 ± 2.8
Hairless mouse skin	0.028 ± 0.002	11.7 ± 0.67

Note: Results are means ± SD for 4 skin specimens.

increase in MGBG epidermal content compared to saline and *N*-methylpyrrolidone vehicle (Table 55).

3. Methotrexate

Effectiveness of systemically administered methotrexate (MTX) in severe recalcitrant psoriasis has prompted attempts to treat the disease by topical application of the drug. Topical therapy, however, is generally ineffective clinically.[198] Lack of percutaneous penetration has been suggested to explain the ineffectiveness of topically applied MTX. However, quantitative estimates of percutaneously absorbed MTX vary.[199] Ball et al.[199] used Vehicle N and observed increased penetration of methotrexate (MTX) on human skin. Comparison was made of permeation from a water and *n*-decylmethyl sulfoxide vehicle (Table 56). Comaish and Juhlin[200] recovered 0.07 to 0.5% of the total applied dose (approximately 1 mg) in the urine of four patients treated topically with MTX. Newbold and Stoughton[201] reported in vitro penetration of 3 to 16% of the total applied dose (0.5 to 32 μg) through hairless mouse skin and human skin. The larger percentages reported by Newbold and Stoughton reflect the smaller total amount applied in their experiments. McCullough et al.[202] reported cumulative penetration after 20 hr of only 0.001 to 0.004% from topical application of aqueous solutions containing 0.05 to 2% MTX.

Wallace et al.[203] studied the penetration of MTX through hairless mouse and human skin in vitro. At pH 8.2, 0.05% of the total applied dose of MTX (1 mg/0.4 mℓ) penetrated within a 30-hr period. Although flux through human skin varied more than through mouse skin, the average penetration rates and lag times were not significantly different (Table 57).

Table 58
CUMULATIVE PERCENT
PENETRATION OF 5-
FLUOROURACIL[204]

| Time | Human skin | | Mouse skin | |
	LSC[a]	GLC[b]	LSC[a]	GLC[b]
30 min	1.2	1.5	1.1	1.5
1 hr	1.3	2.2	1.8	2.0
2 hr	2.0	2.6	2.9	2.6
3 hr	2.7	3.4	5.4	3.8
6 hr	4.0	3.0	8.5	11.7
16 hr	8.3	5.7	16.7	19.7
24 hr	12.9	6.1	22.6	30.6

Note: 0.02 mℓ of a 4% solution was applied to the
epidermis. All human samples were from ad-
jacent areas of the same leg. All values represent a mean of four samples.

[a]   Liquid scintillation counting.
[b]   Gas liquid chromatography.

Table 59
MEAN 20-HR PENETRATION DATA OF 5-FLUOROURACIL[204]

| Samples | Human skin | | Mouse skin | |
	LSC (%)	GLC (%)	LSC (%)	GLC (%)
1	4.3	6.7	23.1	43.0
2	11.3	11.2	11.2	16.4
3	13.1	12.0	33.1	17.3
4	28.1	6.4	26.5	13.5
5	5.3	7.9	32.1	39.7
6	17.2	19.3	—	—
7	6.3	6.7	—	—
8	7.2	13.5	—	—
9	—	40.1	—	—
Mean ± SD	11.6 ± 7.5	13.4 ± 10.1	25.2 ± 7.9	25.9 ± 12.6

Note: 0.01 mℓ of a 4% solution was applied to the epidermis. Samples 1—4 were
from one leg; samples 5—9 were from another leg.

4. 5-Fluorouracil (FU)

Topical application of 5-fluorouracil has proved to be a valuable treatment of various
diseases including actinic keratoses, various epithelial neoplasms, and psoriasis. Cohen and
Stoughton[204] studied penetration of 5-fluorouracil through human and hairless mouse skin
in vitro (Table 58).

Table 59 compares the penetration of 0.01 mℓ of a 4% solution applied to 8 human skins
and 5 mouse samples after 20 hr. For comparative purposes with other molecules, Table 60
expresses the mean 20-hr data as molar transepidermal fluxes of FU per unit time. The drug
is most often administered topically in the form of 1 to 5% solutions in propylene glycol
since this vehicle is known to effectively increase the skin penetration of various topical
drugs.[205,206]

Table 60
MEAN 20-HR SAMPLES EXPRESSED AS
FLUX PER UNIT TIME OF 5-
FLUOROURACIL[204]

Sample	Method	Flux[a] mol/cm²/hr
Human skin	Liquid scintillation	1.09×10^{-8}
Human skin	Gas chromatographic	1.26×10^{-8}
Mouse skin	Liquid scintillation	2.37×10^{-8}
Mouse skin	Gas chromatographic	2.44×10^{-8}

Note: Mean 20-hr data from Table 2.

[a] Skin area exposed to drug was 1.63 cm².

The results indicate fairly high penetration of FU through excised human and hairless mouse skin. The rate of penetration of FU was of the same order of magnitude in both species, but the total penetration was significantly higher in the mouse skin samples. The percent penetration is of the same order of magnitude as that calculated by Dillaha[207] from urinary excretion data following topical application of FU on five patients. He had calculated a 10 to 15% penetration which agrees well with values of 13 and 11%.[204]

Mollgaard et al.[208] compared the permeation characteristics of two prodrug esters of 5-FU with the parent compound using excised human skin. The comparative cumulative permeation profiles show that the 1-butyryloxymethyl derivative (II) of 5-fluorouracil penetrates the skin at a rate about five times faster than that of 5-fluorouracil, while the 1-pivaloyloxymethyl derivative (III) is absorbed at a rate about two times faster. These differences in skin permeation rest certainly on the different physicochemical characteristics of the compound. The derivatives II and III are more lipophilic than 5-fluorouracil as expressed in terms of partition coefficients between octanol and water. Due to the increased lipophilicity, the derivatives might penetrate the lipoidal stratum corneum more readily. Although having the highest lipophilicity, however, the derivative III showed a lower rate of permeation than compound II which means that factors other than lipophilicity are important, e.g., drug-vehicle interactions.

The results of this study demonstrate that *N*-acyloxy-methyl derivatives of 5-fluorouracil may be promising prodrug candidates with the purpose of providing a more efficient topical delivery of the parent drug. This conclusion is especially evident on the basis of the results obtained with the butyryloxymethyl derivative in that this compound permeates about five times more readily through the human skin than 5-fluorouracil and at the same time is delivered completely in the form of the parent drug due to extensive cutaneous metabolism.

5. Vidarabine

Yu et al.[209] studied the percutaneous behavior of vidarabine (9-β-D-arabinofuranosylad-enine, I) in hairless mouse skin. Experiments with *n*-pentanol were included to determine any possible effects of molecular size. Comparison of the permeability coefficients of I in the various membrane preparations revealed that stripped skin was ~ 100 times more permeable than full thickness skin, while the dermis was >1000 times more permeable. A similar relationship also existed for the permeation of *n*-pentanol, but the permeability differences were much smaller. This evidence suggests that, while the stratum corneum is the major diffusional barrier, the epidermis may be significantly less permeable than the dermis (Table 61).

Table 61
PERMEABILITY COEFFICIENTS OF I AND *n*-PENTANOL IN VARIOUS COMPONENTS OF HAIRLESS MOUSE SKIN[209]

	Permeability coefficients, cm/sec	
Stratum	**1**	**1**
Stratum corneum	3.00×10^{-8}	3.85×10^{-6}
Epidermis	4.14×10^{-6}	2.71×10^{-5}
Dermis	3.83×10^{-5}	7.51×10^{-5}

Table 62
PENETRATION OF ACYCLOVIR THROUGH GUINEA PIG SKINS IN VITRO[210]

Exp. no.	Drug/vehicle	Lag time (hr)[a]	Flux (μg/cm$^2 \cdot$ hr)[b]
1	5% ACV/PEG	65	.182
2	5% ACV/PEG	77	.165
3	5% ACV/PEG	37	.068
4	0.5% ACV/DMSO	14	.676
5	0.5% ACV/DMSO	—	.438
6	0.5% ACV/DMSO	—	.284
7	0.5% ACV/DMSO	12	.432

[a] Time between beginning of the experiment and the intercept of the slope on the x-axis in a plot of drug concentration in the receiver chamber (y) vs. time (x).

[b] Flux was calculated from the steady-state slope of plots of drug concentration vs. time, the area of the skin surface exposed to drug, and the volume of the receiver chamber.

6. Acyclovir

Spruance et al.[210] measured the penetration of acyclovir (ACV) through guinea pig skin in vitro from different drug vehicles and compared these findings with the efficacy of two topical formulations of the drug in the treatment of an experimental cutaneous herpes simplex virus infection. ACV is a potent new compound with striking in vitro activity against herpes simplex virus (Table 62). The mean flux of 5% ACV from PEG in three experiments was 0.14 ± 0.06 in DMSO. A higher concentration of ACV in DMSO would have a proportionately higher flux. In addition, the onset of detectable ACV in the receiver chamber (lag time) occurred more quickly when DMSO was the vehicle.

The penetration of ACV through guinea pig skin in vitro was markedly greater with DMSO than when PEG was the vehicle. When 5% ACV in DMSO was compared with 5% ACV in PEG in the treatment of experimental herpes infection in the guinea pig, ACV/DMSO was more effective. The effectiveness of antivirals in DMSO in the guinea pig is likely related to drug penetration and development of a means to enhance delivery of antivirals to the target cells would appear to be a potentially fruitful next step to further the effectiveness of topical antiherpes virus therapy in humans.

7. Mercaptopurine

Sloan et al.[211] studied prodrug alkylated derivatives of 6-mercaptopurine, its riboside, and 2-amino-6-mercaptopurine riboside. They evaluated the delivery of the thiopurines through the skin of hairless mice. The pivaloyloxymethyl derivatives showed the greatest potential for enhancing the penetration of the thiopurines, delivering 5 to 13 times more 6-mercaptopurine itself.

8. Hallucinogenic Agents

Bailey and Briggs[212] investigated the percutaneous absorption of phencyclidine hydrochloride, a widely abused hallucinogenic drug in intact hairless mouse skin. Four hours after topical application, the mean phencyclidene concentration in the livers was 1730 ng/g.

REFERENCES

1. **Katz, M. and Poulsen, B. J.,** Absorption of drugs through the skin, *Handbook of Experimental Pharmacology,* Brodie, B. B. and Gillette, J., Eds., Springer-Verlag, Berlin, 1971, 104.
2. **Reiss, F.,** Percutaneous absorption, a critical and historical review, *Am. J. Med. Sci.,* 252, 588, 1966.
3. **Tregear, R. T.,** The permeability of skin to molecules of widely-differing properties, *Progress In The Biological Sciences In Relation to Dermatology,* Vol. 2. Rook, A. and Champion, R. H., Eds., Cambridge University Press, London, 1964, 275.
4. **Winkelmann, R. K.,** The relationship of the structure of the epidermis to percutaneous absorption, *Br. J. Dermatol.,* 81(Suppl. 4), 11, 1969.
5. **Marzulli, F. N.,** Barriers to skin penetration, *J. Invest. Dermatol.,* 39, 387, 1962.
6. **Lindsey, D.,** *Percutaneous Penetration, Proceedings of the XII International Congress Of Dermatology,* Pillsbury, D. M. and Livingood, C. S., Eds., Excerpta Medica, Amsterdam, 1963, 407.
7. **Wester, R. C. and Maibach, H. I.,** Relationship of topical dose and percutaneous absorption in rhesus monkey and man, *J. Invest. Dermatol.,* 67, 518, 1976.
8. **Poulsen, B. J.,** *Design Of Topical Drug Products: Biopharmaceutics, Drug Design,* Vol., 4 Ariens, E. J., Ed., Academic Press, New York, 1973, 149.
9. **Bartek, M. J., Labudde, J. A., and Maibach, H. I.,** Skin permeability in vivo: comparison in rat, rabbit, pig, and man, *J. Invest. Dermatol.,* 58, 114, 1972.
10. **Tregear, R. T.,** *Physical Function Of The Skin,* Academic Press, New York, 1966.
11. **Franz, T. J.,** Percutaneous absorption. On the relevance of in vitro data, *J. Invest. Dermatol.,* 64, 190, 1975.
12. **Bronaugh, R. L., Stewart, R. F., Congdon, E. R., and Giles, A. L.,** Methods for in vitro percutaneous absorption studies. I. Comparison with in vivo results, *Toxicol. Appl. Pharmacol.,* 62, 474, 1982.
13. **Wester, R. C. and Maibach, H. I.,** Cutaneous pharmacokinetics: 10 steps to percutaneous absorption, *Drug. Metab. Rev.,* 14, 169, 1983.
14. **Barry, B. W.,** *Dermatological Formulations,* Marcel Decker, New York, 1983.
15. **Flynn, G. L.,** Topical drug absorption and topical pharmaceutical systems, in *Modern Pharmaceutics,* Barker, G. S. and Rhodes, C. T., Eds., Marcel Decker, New York, 1979.
16. **Idson, B.,** Vehicle effects in percutaneous absorption, *Drug Metab. Rev.,* 14, 207, 1983.
17. **McKenzie, A. W.,** Percutaneous absorption of steroids, *Arch. Dermatol.,* 86, 611, 1962.
18. **McKenzie, A. W. and Stoughton, R. B.,** Method for comparing percutaneous absorption of steroids, *Arch. Dermatol.,* 86, 608, 1962.
19. **Moore-Robinson, M. and Christie, G. A.,** Vasoconstrictor activity of topical corticosteroids-methodology and results, *Br. J. Dermatol.,* 82 (Suppl. 6), 86, 1970.
20. **McKenzie, A. W.,** Comparison of steroids by vasoconstriction, *Br. J. Dermatol.,* 78, 182, 1966.
21. **Reid, J. and Brooke, D. B.,** Topical corticosteroids — an experimental evaluation of the vasoconstrictor test as an index of antiinflammatory activity, *Br. J. Dermatol.,* 80, 328, 1968.
22. **Baker, J. and Sattar, H. A.,** The assessment of four new fluocortolone analogues by a modified vasoconstriction assay, *Br. J. Dermatol.,* 80, 46, 1968.
23. **Kligman, A. M.,** Topical pharmacology and toxicology of dimethyl-sulfoxide, *JAMA,* 193, 796, 1965.
24. **Fredriksson, T.,** Studies on the percutaneous absorption of parathion and paraoxon. II. Distribution of ^{32}P-labelled parathion within the skin, *Acta Derm. Venereol.,* 41, 344, 1961.
25. **Fredriksson, T.,** Influence of solvents and surface active agents on the barrier function of the skin towards sarin. I. Development of method, *Acta Derm. Venereol.,* 43, 91, 1963.

26. **Nabb, D. P., Stein, W. J., and Hayes, W. J., Jr.,** Rate Of Skin Absorption Of Parathion And Paraoxon, *Arch. Environ. Health,* 12, 501, 1966.
27. **Vickers, C. F. H.,** Percutaneous absorption of sodium fusidate and fusidic acid, *Br. J. Dermatol.,* 81, 902, 1969.
28. **Grasso, P. and Landsdown, A. B. G.,** Methods of measuring, and factors affecting percutaneous absorption, *J. Soc. Cosmet. Chem.,* 23, 481, 1972.
29. **Higuchi, T.,** *Design Of Biopharmaceutical Properties Through Prodrugs And Analogs,* Roche, E. B., Ed., American Pharmaceutical Association, Washington, D.C., 1977, 409.
30. **Rytting, H., Davis, S. S., and Higuchi, T.,** *J. Pharm. Sci.,* 61, 817, 1972.
31. **Higuchi, T. and Davis, S. S.,** *J. Pharm. Sci.,* 59, 1376, 1970.
32. **Blank, I. H.,** Penetration of low-molecular weight alcohols into skin. I. Effect of concentration of alcohol and type of vehicle, *J. Invest. Dermatol.,* 43, 415, 1964.
33. **Scheuplein, R. J.,** Mechanism of percutaneous absorption. I. Routes of penetration and the influence of solubility, *J. Invest. Dermatol.,* 45, 334, 1965.
34. **Scheuplein, R. J.,** Mechanism of percutaneous absorption. II. Transient diffusion and the relative importance of various routes of skin penetration, *J. Invest. Dermatol.,* 48, 79, 1967.
35. **Scheuplein, R. and Ross, L.,** Mechanisms of percutaneous absorption. V. Percutaneous absorption of solvent deposited solids, *J. Invest. Dermatol.,* 62, 353, 1974.
36. **Scheuplein, R. J. and Blank, I. H.,** Mechanisms of percutaneous absorption. IV. Penetration of non-electrolytes (alcohols) from aq. soln. and from pure liquids, *J. Invest. Dermatol.,* 60, 286, 1973.
37. **Scheuplein, R. J. and Ross, L. W.,** Mechanisms of percutaneous absorption. I. Percutaneous absorption of solvent deposited solids, *J. Invest. Dermatol.,* 62, 353, 1974.
38. **Scheuplein, R. J. and Blank, I. H.,** Permeability of the skin, *Physiol. Rev.,* 51, 702, 1971.
39. **Scheuplein, R. J. and Ross, L.,** Effects of surfactants and solvents on the permeability of epidermis, *J. Soc. Cosmet. Chem.,* 21, 853, 1970.
40. **Baker, H and Kligman, A. M.,** Measurement of transepidermal water loss by electrical hygrometry, *Arch. Dermatol.,* 96, 441, 1967.
41. **Blank, I. H.,** Further observations on factors which influence the water content of the stratum corneum, *J. Invest. Dermatol.,* 21, 259, 1953.
42. **Davies, J.T. and Rideal, E. K.,** *Interfacial Phenomena,* Academic Press, New York, 1963, 154.
43. **Durrheim, H., Flynn, G. L., Higuchi, W. I., and Behl, C. R.,** Permeation of hairless mouse skin. I. Experimental methods and comparison with human epidermal permeation by alkanols, *J. Pharm. Sci.,* 69, 781, 1980.
44. **Flynn, G. L., Durrheim, H., and Higuchi, W. I.,** Permeation of hairless mouse skin. II. Membrane sectioning techniques and influence on alkanol permeability, *J. Pharm. Sci.,* 70, 52, 1981.
45. **Behl, C. R., Flynn, G. L., Kurihara, T., Harper, N., Smith, W., Higuchi, W. I., Ho, N. F. H., and Pierson, C. L.,** Hydration and percutaneous absorption. I. Influence of hydration on alkanol penetration through hairless mouse skin, *J. Invest. Dermatol.,* 75, 346, 1980.
46. **Behl, C. R., Bellantone, N. H., and Pei, J.,** Effects of the Alkyl Chain Length and Anatomical Site on the Alkanol Permeability Through Fuzzy Rat Skins, Basic Pharmaceutics Abstract 10, presented at the 130th Annual Meeting of A.Ph.A., New Orleans, La., April 9, 1983.
47. **Behl, C. R. and Bellantone, N. H.,** Influence of the Alkyl Chain Length on the In-Situ Permeation of N-Alkanols Through the Fuzzy Rat Skins and Comparison with the In-Vitro Data. Comparisons of the Fuzzy Rat and the Hairless Mouse Skin Results, Basic Pharmaceutics Abstract 38, presented at the 31st National Meeting of the A.P.S., Miami Beach, Fla., November 14, 1983.
48. **Behl, C. R., Meyer, R., and Flynn, G. L.,** Percutaneous Absorption by the Living Mouse. Uptake of Water and N-Alkanols Across Normal and Stripped Skins, Basic Pharmaceutics Abstract 22, presented at the 128th Annual Meeting of the American Pharmaceutical Association, St. Louis, Mo., April 1981.
49. **Meyer, R., Behl, C. R., and Flynn, G. L.,** Permeation of Hairless Mouse Skin. V. Further Observations on the Influence of Adhesive Tape Stripping. Basic Pharmaceutics Abstract 13, presented At The 128th Annual Meeting Of The A.Ph.A., St. Louis, Mo., April, 1981.
50. **Behl, C. R., Barrett, M., Flynn, G. L., Kurihara, T., Walters, K. A., Gatmaitan, O. G., Harper, N., Higuchi, W. I., Ho, N. F. H., and Pierson, C. L.,** Hydration and percutaneous absorption influences of stripping and scalding on hydration alterations of the permeability of hairless mouse skin to water and N-alkanols, *J. Pharm. Sci.,* 71, 229, 1982.
51. **Behl, C. R.,** Systems Approach To The Study Of Vaginal Drug Absorption In The Rhesus Monkey, Ph.D. thesis, University of Michigan, Ann Arbor, 1979.
52. **Liron, Z. and Cohen, S.,** Percutaneous absorption of alkanoic acids. I. A study of operational conditions, *J. Pharm. Sci.,* 73, 534, 1984.
53. **Liron, Z. and Cohen, S.,** Percutaneous absorption of alkanoic acids. II. Application of regular solution theory, *J. Pharm. Sci.,* 73, 538, 1984.

54. **Behl, C. R. and Flynn, G. L.,** Permeability of hairless mouse skin to *N*-alkanoic acids, unpublished data.
55. **Hoelgaard, A. and Molgaard, B.,** Permeation of linoleic acid through skin in vitro, *J. Pharm. Pharmacol.,* 34, 610, 1982.
56. **Stoughton, R. B. and Fritsch, W.,** Influence of DMSO on human percutaneous absorption, *Arch. Dermatol.,* 90, 512, 1964.
57. **Sekura, D. L. and Scala, J.,** in *Advances in Biology Of Skin,* Vol. 12, Montagna, W., Stoughton, R. B. and Van Scott, E. J., Eds., Appleton-Century-Crofts, New York, 1972, 257.
58. **Nacht, S., Yeung, D., Beasley, J. N., Anjo, M. D., and Maibach, H. I.,** Benzoyl peroxide: percutaneous penetration and metabolic disposition, *J. Am. Acad. Dermatol.,* 4, 31, 1981.
59. **Holzmann, H., Morsches, B., and Benes, P.,** The absorption of benzoyl peroxide from leg ulcers, *Arzneim. Forsch.,* 29, 1180, 1979.
60. **Karim, A.,** Transdermal absorption: a unique opportunity for constant delivery of nitroglycerin, *Drug Dev. Ind. Pharm.,* 9, 671, 1983.
61. **Armstrong, P. W., Armstrong, J. A., and Marks, G. S.,** Blood levels after sublingual nitroglycerin, *Circulation,* 59, 585, 1979.
62. **McNiff, E. F., Yacobi, A., Young-Chang, F. M., Golden, L. H., Goldfarb, A., and Fung, H. L.,** Nitroglycerin phamacokinetics after intravenous infusion in normal subjects, *J. Pharm. Sci.,* 70, 1054, 1981.
63. **Mintz, G. S.,** *Selected Readings,* Biomedical Information, New York, 1977.
64. **Nickerson, M.,** in *The Pharmacological Basis Of Therapeutics,* Goodman, L. S. and Gilman, A., Eds., MacMillan, New York 1970, 751.
65. **Chien, Y., Keshary, P., Huang, Y., and Sarpotdar, P.,** Comparative controlled skin permeation of nitroglycerin from marketed transdermal delivery system, *J. Pharm. Sci.,* 72, 968, 1983.
66. **Keshary, P. K.,** Mechanism Of Transdermal Controlled Nitroglycerin Administration — Control of Skin Permeation Rate And Optimization, Ph.D. thesis, The State University of Rutgers, New Brunswick, N. J., 1984.
67. **Michaels, A. S., Chandrasekcaran, S. K., and Shaw, J. E.,** Drug permeation through human skin: theory and in vitro experimental measurements, *A. I. Ch. E. J.,* 21, 985, 1975.
68. **Bronaugh, R. L., Congdon, E. R., and Scheuplein, R. J.,** The effect of cosmetic vehicle on the penetration of *N*-nitrosodiethanolamine through excised human skin, *J. Invest. Dermatol.,* 76, 94, 1981.
69. **Marzulli, F. N., Callahan, J. F., and Brown, D. W. C.,** Chemical structure and penetrating capacity of a short series of organic phosphates and phosphoric acid, *J. Invest. Dermatol.,* 44, 339, 1965.
70. **Dempski, R. E., Portnoff, J. B., and Wase, A. W.,** In vitro release and in vivo penetration studies of a topical steroid from nonaqueous vehicles, *J. Pharm. Sci.,* 58, 579, 1969.
71. **Black, J. B. and Howes, D.,** *J. Soc. Cosmet. Chem.,* 26, 205, 1975.
72. **Calensnick, B., Costello, C. H., Ryan, J. P., and DiGregorio, G. J.,** *Toxicol. Appl. Pharmacol.,* 32, 204, 1975.
73. **Brown, D. W. C. and Ulsamer, A. G.,** *Food Cosmet. Toxicol.,* 13, 81, 1975.
74. **Bye, P. G. T., Morison, W., and Rhodes, E. L.,** *Br. J. Dermatol.,* 93, 209, 1975.
75. **Croshaw, B.,** *J. Soc. Cosmet. Chem.,* 28, 3, 1977.
76. **Smith, G. M. and Peck, G. E.,** *J. Pharm. Sci.,* 65, 727, 1976.
77. **Schorr, W. D. and Mohajerin, A. H.,** *Arch. Dermatol.,* 93, 721, 1966.
78. **Marzulli, F. N. and Maibach, H. I.,** *J. Soc. Cosmet. Chem.,* 24, 399, 1973.
79. **Komatsu, H. and Suzuki, M.,** Percutaneous absorption of butylparaben through guinea pig skin in vitro, *J. Pharm. Sci.,* 68, 596, 1979.
80. **Albery, J. W. and Hadgraft, J.,** Percutaneous absorption: in vivo experiments, *J. Pharm. Pharmacol.,* 31, 140, 1979.
81. **Albery, W. J., Guy, R. H., and Hadgraft, J.,** Percutaneous absorption: transport in the dermis, *Int. J. Pharm.,* 15, 125, 1983.
82. **Stoughton, R. B., Clendenning, W. E., and Kruse, D.,** Percutaneous absorption of nicotinic acid and derivatives, *J. Invest. Dermatol.,* 35, 337, 1960.
83. **Fountain, R. B., Baker, B. S., Hadgraft, J. W., and Sarkany, I.,** The rate of absorption and duration of action of four different solutions of methyl nicotinate, *Br. J. Dermatol.,* 81, 202, 1969.
84. **Henschel, V. and Jaminet, F.,** *J. Pharm. Belg.,* 27, 743, 1972.
85. **Fulton, G. P., Farber, E. M., and Moreci, A. P.,** *J. Invest. Dermatol.,* 33, 317, 1959.
86. **Guy, R. H. and Maibach, H. I.,** Rapid radial transport of methyl nicotinate in the dermis, *Arch. Dermatol. Res.,* 273, 91, 1982.
87. **Sweeney, T. M., Downes, A. M., and Matoltsy, A. B.,** The effect of dimethylsulfoxide on the epidermal water barrier, *J. Invest. Dermatol.,* 46, 300, 1966.
88. **Elfbaum, S. G. and Laden, K.,** The effect of dimethyl sulfoxide on percutaneous absorption: a mechanistic study, part I. *J. Soc. Cosmet. Chem.,* 19, 119, 1968.

89. **Sprott, W. E.,** Surfactants and percutaneous absorption, *Trans. St. John's Hosp. Dermatol. Soc.,* 51, 56, 1965.

90. **Roberts, M. S., Shorey, C. D., Arnold, R., and Anderson, R. A.,** *Aust. J. Pharm. Sci.,* NS3, 81, 1974.

91. **Roberts, M. S. and Anderson, R. A.,** *J. Pharm. Pharmacol.,* 27, 599, 1975.

92. **Roberts, M. S., Anderson, R. A., and Swarbrick, J.,** Permeability of human epidermis to phenolic compounds, *J. Pharm. Pharmacol.,* 29, 677, 1977.

93. **Davis, S. S., Higuchi, T., and Rytting, J. H.,** *Adv. Pharm. Sci.,* 4, 73, 1974.

94. **Hansch, C.,** *in Drug Design,* Vol. 1, Ariens, E. J., Ed., Academic Press, New York, 1971.

95. **Leo, A., Hansch, C., and Elkins, D.,** *Chem. Rev.,* 71, 525, 1971.

96. **Scheuplein, R. J., Blank, I. H., Brauner, G. J., and Macfarlane, D. J.,** Percutaneous absorption of steroids, *J. Invest. Dermatol.,* 52, 63, 1969.

97. **Behl, C. R., Linn, E. E., Flynn, G. L., Pierson, C. L., Higuchi, W. I., and Ho, N. F. H.,** Permeation of skin and eschar by antiseptics. I. Baseline studies with phenol, *J. Pharm. Sci.,* 72, 391, 1983.

98. **Behl, C. R., Linn, E. E., Flynn, G. L., Ho, N. F. H., Higuchi, W. I., and Pierson, C. L.,** Permeation of skin and eschar by antiseptics. II. Influence of controlled burns on the permeation of phenol, *J. Pharm. Sci.,* 72, 397, 1983.

99. **Roberts, M. S., Anderson, R. A., Swarbrick, J., and Moore, D. E.,** The percutaneous absorption of phenolic compounds: the mechanism of diffusion across the stratum cornuem, *J. Pharm. Pharmacol.,* 30, 486, 1978.

100. **Stolar, M. E., Rossi, G. V., Barr, M.,** The effect of various ointment bases on the percutaneous absorption of salicylates I, II, *J. Am. Pharm. Assoc.,* 49, 144, 1960.

101. **Roberts, M. S. and Horlock, E.,** Effect of repeated skin application on percutaneous absorption of salicylic acid, *J. Pharm. Sci.,* 67, 1685, 1978.

102. **Loveday, D. E.,** *J. Soc. Cosmet. Chem.,* 12, 224, 1961.

103. **Gstirnen, F. and Elsner, R.,** *Arzneim. Forsch.,* 14, 281, 1964.

104. **Hlynka, J. N., Anderson, A. J., and Riedel, B. E.,** *Can. J. Pharm. Sci.,* 4, 92, 1969.

105. **Washitake, M., Anmo, T., Tanaka, I., Arita, T., and Nakano, M.,** *J. Pharm. Sci.,* 64, 397, 1975.

106. **Barry, III, H., Marcus, F., and Colaizzi, J. L.,** Value of repeated tests in a percutaneous absorption study, *J. Pharm. Sci.,* 61, 172, 1972.

107. **Arita, T., Hori, R., Anmo, T., Washitake, M., Akatsu, M., and Yajima, T.,** Studies on percutaneous absorption of drugs, *Chem. Pharm. Bull.,* 18, 1045, 1970.

108. **Elias, P. M., Cooper, E. R., Korc, A., and Brown, B. E.,** Percutaneous transport in relation to stratum corneum structure and lipid composition, *J. Invest. Dermatol.,* 76, 297, 1981.

109. **Shen, W. W., Danti, A. G., and Bruscato, F. N.,** Effect on nonionic surfactants on percutaneous absorption of salicylic acid and sodium salicylate in the presence of dimethyl sulfoxide, *J. Pharm. Sci.,* 65, 1780, 1976.

110. **Higuchi, T.,** Physical chemical analyses of percutaneous absorption process from creams and ointments, *J. Soc. Cosmet. Chem.,* 11, 85, 1960.

111. **Maruta, H., Muami, K., Yagamata, T., and Noda, K.,** Percutaneous absorption of methyl salicylate from medicated plaster in mice and humans, *Kurume Med. J.,* 24, 131, 1977.

112. **Feldman, R. and Maibach, H. I.,** Absorption of some organic compounds through the skin in man, *J. Invest. Dermatol.,* 54, 399, 1970.

113. **Loftsson, T. and Bodor, N.,** Improved delivery through biological membranes. X. Percutaneous absorption and metabolism of methylsulfinylmethyl 2-acetoxybenzoate and related aspirin prodrugs, *J. Pharm. Sci.,* 70, 756, 1981.

114. **Fischer, T. and Hartvig, P.,** Skin absorption of 8-hydroxyquinolines, *Lancet,* 1, 603, 1977.

115. **Degen, P. H., Moppert, J., Schmid, K., and Weirich, E. G.,** Percutaneous absorption of clioquinol (Vioform), *Dermatologica,* 159, 295, 1979.

116. **Stohs, J. J., Ezzedeen, F. W., Anderson, K. A., Baldwin, J. N., and Makoid, M. C.,** Percutaneous absorption of idochlorhydroxyquin in humans, *J. Invest. Dermatol.,* 82, 195, 1984.

117. **Kammerau, B., Zesch, A., and Schaefer, H.,** Absolute concentrations of dithranol and triacetyldithranol in the skin layers after local treatment, *J. Invest. Dermatol.,* 64, 145, 1975.

118. **Selim, M. M., Goldberg, L. H., Schaefer, H., Bishop, S. C., and Farbers, E. M.,** Penetration studies on topical anthralin, *Br. J. Dermatol.,* 105 (Suppl. 20), 101, 1981.

119. **Schalla, W., Bauer, E., and Schaefer, H.,** Skin permeability of anthralin, *Br. J. Dermatol.,* 105 (Suppl. 20), 104, 1981.

120. **Zesch, A., Schaefer, H., and Stuttgen, G.,** The quantitative distribution of percutaneously applied caffeine in human skin, *Arch. Dermatol.,* 266, 277, 1979.

121. **Sloan, K. B. and Bodor, N.,** Hydroxylmethyl and acyloxymethyl prodrugs of theophylline: enhanced delivery of polar drugs through skin, *Int. J. Pharm.,* 12, 299, 1982.

122. **Idson, B.,** Percutaneous absorption, *J. Pharm. Sci.,* 64, 901, 1975.
123. **Wurster, D. E., Ostrenga, J. A., and Metheson, L. E.,** Sarin transport across excised human skin. I. Permeability and absorption characteristics, *J. Pharm. Sci.,* 68, 1406, 1979.
124. **Metheson, L. E., Wurster, D. E., and Ostrenga, J. A.,** Sarin transport across excised human skin. II. Effect of solvent pretreatment on permeability, *J. Pharm. Sci.,* 68, 1410, 1979.
125. **Wurster, D. E. and Kramer, S. F.,** Some factors influencing percutaneous absorption, *J. Pharm. Sci.,* 50, 288, 1961.
126. **Treherne, J. E.,** The permeability of skin to some non-electrolytes, *J. Physiol.,* 133, 171, 1956.
127. **Smith, W. M.,** Ph.D. thesis, University of Michigan, Ann Arbor, 1982.
128. **Marzulli, F. N.,** In vivo skin penetration studies of 2,4-toluenediamine, 2,4-diaminoanisole, 2-nitro-*p*-phenylenediamine, *p*-dioxane, and *N*-nitrosodiethanolamine in cosmetics, *Food Cosmet. Toxicol.,* 19, 743, 1981.
129. **Shahi, V. and Zatz, J. L.,** Effect of formulation factors on penetration of hydrocortisone through mouse skin, *J. Pharm. Sci.,* 67, 789, 1978.
130. **Bettley, F. R.,** The influence of soap on the permeability of the epidermis, *Br. J. Dermatol.,* 73, 448, 1961.
131. **Scala, J., McOsker, D. E., and Reeler, H. H.,** The perception of ionic surfactants, *J. Invest. Dermatol.,* 50, 371, 1968.
132. **Howes, D.,** The percutaneous absorption of some anionic surfactants, *J. Soc. Cosmet. Chem.,* 26, 47, 1975.
133. **Blank, I. H. and Gould, E.,** Penetration of anionic surfactants (surface active agents) into skin. I. Penetration of sodium laurate and sodium dodecyl sulfate into excised human skin, *J. Invest. Dermatol.,* 33, 327, 1959.
134. **Emery, G. and Dugard, Ph.H.,** The influence of dimethyl sulphoxide on the percutaneous migration of potassium dodecyl(^{35}S) sulphate, *Br. J. Dermatol.,* 81 (Suppl. 4), 63, 1969.
135. **Bettley, F. R. and Donoghue, E.,** Effect of soap on the diffusion of water through isolated human epidermis, *Nature (London),* 185, 17, 1960.
136. **Aguian, A. J. and Weiner, M. A.,** Percutaneous absorption studies on chloramphenicol solutions, *J. Pharm. Sci.,* 58, 210, 1969.
137. **Blank, I. H. and Gould E.,** Penetration of anionic surfactants into skin. II. Study of mechanisms which impede the penetration of synthetic anionic surfactants into skin, *J. Invest. Dermatol.,* 37, 311, 1961.
138. **Blank, I. H. and Gould, E.,** Penetration of anionic surfactants into skin. III. Penetration from buffered sodium laurate solutions, *J. Invest. Dermatol.,* 37, 485, 1961.
139. **Blank, I. H., Gould, E., and Theobald, A.,** Penetration of cationic surfactants into skin, *J. Invest. Dermatol.,* 42, 363, 1964.
140. **Bettley, F. R.,** The irritant effect of soap in relation to epidermal permeability, *Br. J. Dermatol.,* 75, 113, 1963.
141. **Putnam, F. W.,** The interactions of proteins and synthetic detergents, *Adv. Protein Chem.,* 4, 79, 1948.
142. **Klotz, I. M.,** The nature of some ion-protein complexes, *Cold Spring Harbor Symp.,* 14, 97, 1949.
143. **Chowhan, Z. T. and Pritchard, R.,** Effect of surfactants on percutaneous absorption of naproxen. I. Comparison of rabbit, rat, and human excised skin, *J. Pharm. Sci.,* 67, 1272, 1978.
144. **Lansdown, A. B. and Grasso, P.,** Physico-chemical factors influencing epidermal damage by surface active agents, *Br. J. Dermatol.,* 86, 361, 1972.
145. **Vinson, L. J. and Choman, B. R.,** Percutaneous absorption and surface active agents, *J. Soc. Cosmet. Chem.,* 11, 127, 1960.
146. **Stelzer, J. M., Colaizzi, J. L., and Wurdack, P. J.,** *J. Pharm. Sci.,* 57, 1732, 1968.
147. **Mezei, M. and Ryan, K.,** *J. Pharm. Sci.,* 61, 1329, 1972.
148. **Block, L. H. and Gupta, S. K.,** Percutaneous transport of antihistamines, *J. Soc. Cosmet. Chem.,* 30, 157, 1984.
148a. **Mishiyama, T. and Mitsui, T.,** In-vivo percutaneous absorption of polyoxyethylene lauryl ether in hairless mice, *J. Soc. Cosmet. Chem.,* 34, 263, 1983.
149. **Bettley, F. R.,** The influence of detergents and surfactants on epidermal permeability, *Br. J. Dermatol.,* 77, 98, 1965.
150. **Dalvi, U. G. and Zatz, J. L.,** Effect of nonionic surfactants on penetration of dissolved benzocaine through hairless mouse skin, *J. Soc. Cosmet. Chem.,* 32, 87, 1981.
151. **Dalvi, U. G. and Zatz, J. L.,** Effect of skin binding on percutaneous transport of benzocaine from aqueous suspensions and solutions, *J. Pharm. Sci.,* 71, 824, 1982.
152. **Chowhan, Z. T., Pritchard, R., Rooks, W. H., and Tomolonis, A.,** Effect of surfactants on percutaneous absorption; *in-vivo* and *in-vitro* correlations, *J. Pharm. Sci.,* 67, 1645, 1978.
153. **Tregear, R. T.,** The permeability of skin to albumin dextrans and polyvinyl pyrrolidone, *J. Invest. Dermatol.,* 46, 24, 1966.

154. **Kastin, A. J., Arimura, A., and Schally, A. V.,** Topical absorption of polypeptides with dimethylsulphoxide, *Arch. Dermatol.*, 93, 471, 1966.

155. **Bronaugh, R. L., Stewart, R. F., and Congdon, E. R.,** Methods for *in-vitro* percutaneous absorption studies. II. Animal models for human skin, *Toxicol. Appl. Pharmacol.*, 62, 481, 1982.

156. **Franz, J. M., Gaillard, A., Maibach, H. I., and Schweitzer, A.,** Percutaneous absorption of griseoflulvin and proquazone in the rat and in isolated human skin, *Arch. Dermatol. Res.*, 271, 275, 1981.

157. **Rougier, A., Dupuis, D., Lotti, C., Rouget, R., and Schaefer, H.,** *In-vivo* correlation between stratum corneum reservoir function and percutaneous absorption, *J. Invest. Dermatol.*, 81, 275, 1983.

158. **Feldman, R. J. and Maibach, H. I.,** Percutaneous penetration of steroids in man, *J. Invest. Dermatol.*, 52, 89, 1969.

159. **Malkinson, F. D. and Rothman, S.,** Percutaneous absorption, Handbuch der Haut und Geschlecht Skrauberten Normale und Pathologische der Haut, Vol 1, (Part 1), Erganzungswerk Bd $^1/_3$, Marchionini, A. and Spier, H. W., Eds., Springer Verlag, Berlin, 1963, 90.

160. **Tregear, R. T.,** Molecular movement, the permeability of skin in *Theoretical and Experimental Biology — Physical Functions of Skin*, Academic Press, London, 1966, 1.

161. **Andersen, K.E., Maibach, H. I., and Anjio, M. D.,** The guinea pig: an animal for human skin absorption of hydrocortisone, testosterone, and benzoic acid?, *Br. J. Dermatol.*, 102, 447, 1980.

162. **Stoughton, R. B.,** Animal models for *in-vitro* percutaneous absorption, *Animal Models in Dermatology*, Maibach, H. I., Ed., Churchill Livingstone, Edinburgh, 1975, 121.

163. **Wester, R. C. and Maibach, H. I.,** Rhesus monkey as an animal model for percutaneous absorption, *Animal Models in Dermatology*, Maibach, H. I., Ed., Churchill Livingstone, Edinburgh, 1975, 133.

164. **Galey, W. R., Lonsdale, H. K., and Nacht, S.,** The *in-vitro* permeability of skin and buccal mucosa to selected drugs and tritiated water, *J. Invest. Dermatol.*, 67, 713, 1976.

165. **National Cancer Institute,** Internal reports, Carcinogenesis Technical Report Series, No. 169, Bethesda, Md., 1979.

166. **Maibach, H. I. and Wolfran, L. J.,** Percutaneous penetration of hair dyes, *J. Soc. Cosmet. Chem.*, 32, 223, 1981.

167. **Tregear, R. T.,** The permeability of mammalian skin to ions, *J. Invest. Dermatol.*, 46, 16, 1966.

168. **Friberg, L., Skog, E., and Wahlberg, J. E.,** Resorption of mercuric chloride and methyl mercury dicyandiamide in guinea-pigs through normal skin and through skin pretreated with acetone, alkylarylsulphonate and soap, *Acta Derm. Venereol.*, 41, 40, 1961.

169. **Wahlberg, J. E. and Skog, E.,** The percutaneous absorption of sodium chromate (^{51}Cr) in the guinea pig, *Acta Derm. Venereol.*, 43, 103, 1963.

170. **Blank, I. H. and Scheuplein, R. J.,** The epidermal barrier, in *Progress In The Biological Sciences In Relation To Dermatology*, 2nd ed., Rook, A. J. and Champion, R. H., Eds., Cambridge University Press, London, 1964.

171. **Monash, S.,** Topical anaesthesia of the unbroken skin, *Arch. Dermatol.*, 76, 752, 1957.

172. **Monash, S.,** Location of the superficial barrier to skin penetration, *J. Invest. Dermatol.*, 29, 367, 1957.

173. **Dalili, H. and Adriani, J.,** The efficacy of local anaesthetics in blocking the sensation of itch, burning and pain in normal and "sunburned" skin, *Clin. Pharmacol. Ther.*, 12, 913, 1971.

174. **Akerman, B., Haegerstam, G., Pring, B. G., and Sandberg, R.,** Penetration enhancers and other factors governing percutaneous local anaesthesia with lidocaine, *Acta Pharmacol. Toxicol.*, 45, 58, 1979.

175. **Munro, D. and Stoughton, R.,** Dimethylacetamide (DMAC) and dimethylformamide (DMFA). Effect on percutaneous absorption, *Arch. Dermatol.*, 92, 585, 1965.

176. **Munro, D. D.,** The relationship between percutaneous absorption and stratum corneum retention, *Br. J. Dermatol.*, 81, (Suppl. 4), 92, 1969.

177. **Creasey, N. H., Allenby, A. C., and Schock, C.,** Mechanism of action of accelerants. The effect of cutaneously applied penetration accelerants on the skin circulation of the rat, *Br. J. Dermatol.*, 85, 368, 1971.

178. **Hucker, H. B. and Hoffmann, E. A.,** *J. Pharm. Sci.*, 60, 1049, 1971.

179. **Emori, H. W., Champion, G. D., Bluestone, R., and Paulus, H. E.,** *Ann. Rheum. Dis.*, 32, 433, 1973.

180. **Ishihama, H., Kimata, H., and Mizuschima, Y.,** Percutaneous penetration of indomethacin, *Experimentia*, 35, 798, 1979.

181. **Kyuki, K.,** *Folia Pharmacol. Jpn.*, 79, 461, 1982.

182. **Shima, K., Matsusaka, C., Hirose, M., Noguchi, T., Noguchi, T., and Yamahira, Y.,** Biopharmaceutical characteristics of indomethacia gel ointment, *Chem. Pharm. Bull.*, 29, 2338, 1981.

183. **Panse, P., Zeiller, P., and Sensch, K. H.,** *Arzneim. Forsch.*, 21, 1605, 1971.

184. **Panse, P., Zeiller, P., and Sensch, K. H.,** *Arzneim. Forsch.*, 24, 1298, 1974.

185. **Jackle, H. G.,** *Dtsch. Med. J.*, 23, 245, 1972.

186. **Hwang, C. C. and Danti, A. G.,** Percutaneous absorption of flufenamic acid in rabbits: effect of dimethyl sulfoxide and various nonionic surface-active agents, *J. Pharm. Sci.*, 72, 857, 1983.

187. **Schaefer, H. and Stuettgen, G.,** Penetration of non-steroidal anti-inflammatory (drug) into human skin *in-vitro* and *in-vivo*. Tissue concentrations and flow rates of *p*-butoxyphenylaceto-hydroxamic acid, *Arzneim. Forsch.*, 28, 1021, 1978.

188. **Schiantarelli, P., Cadel, S., Acerbi, D., and Pavesi, L.,** Antiinflammatory activity and bioavailability of percutaneous piroxicam, *Arzneim. Forsch.*, 32, 230, 1982.

189. **Lutzky, B. N., Berkenkopf, J., Ferandez, J., Monahan, M., and Watnick, A. S.,** *Arzneim. Forsch.*, 29 (Suppl. 2), 992, 1979.

190. **Glenn, E. M., Bowman, B. J., and Rohloff, N. A.,** Agents. Actions, 8, 497, 1978.

191. **Maider, S. A.,** Treatment of atopic eczema in children: clinical trial of 10% sodium cromoglycate ointment, *Br. Med. J.*, 1, 1570, 1977.

192. **Bodor, N., Zupan, J., and Selk, S.,** Improved delivery through biological membranes. VII. Dermal delivery of cromoglycic acid (cromolyn) via its prodrugs, *Int. J. Pharm.*, 7, 63, 1980.

193. **Walt, R. P., Kalman, C. J., Hunt, R. H., and Misiewicz, J. J.,** Effect of transdermally administered hyoscin methobromide on nocturnal acid secretion in patients with duodenal ulcer, *Br. Med. J.*, 284, 1736, 1982.

194. **Shaw, J. E. and Chandrasekaran, S. K.,** Controlled topical delivery of drugs for systemic action, *Drug Metab. Rev.*, 8, 223, 1978.

195. **Zackheim, H. S., Karasek, M. A., and Cox, A. J.,** Topical hydroxyurea and psoriasis, *J. Invest. Dermatol.*, 58, 24, 1972.

196. **Shrewsbury, R. P., Foster, T. S., Dittert, L. W., Quigley, J. W., and Leavell, U. W.,** Percutaneous absorption of hydroxyurea through psoriatic lesions, *Curr. Ther. Res. Clin. Exp.*, 28, 1002, 1980.

197. **McCullough, J. L., Weinstein, G. D., Rosenblum, M. G.,and Jenkins, J.,** Percutaneous penetration of methylglyoxal *bis*(guanylhydrazone): effects on hairless mouse epidermis *in-vivo*, *J. Invest. Dermatol.*, 81, 388, 1983.

198. **Stewart, W., Wallace, S., and Ruinikis, J.,** Absorption and local action of methotrexate in human and mouse skin, *Arch. Dermatol.*, 106, 357, 1972.

199. **Ball, M. A., McCullough, J. L., and Weinstein, G.,** Percutaneous absorption of methotrexate: effect on epidermal DNA synthesis in hairless mouse, *J. Invest. Dermatol.,*. 79, 7, 1982.

200. **Comaish, S. and Juhlin, L.,** Site of action of methotrexate in psoriasis, *Arch. Dermatol.*, 100, 99, 1969.

201. **Newbold, P. C. and Stoughton, R. B.,** *J. Invest. Dermatol.*, 58, 319, 1972.

202. **McCullough, J. L., Snyder, D. S., Weinstein, G. D., Friedland, A., and Stein, B.,** Factors affecting human percutaneous penetration of methatrexate and its analogues *in-vitro*, *J. Invest. Dermatol.*, 66, 103, 1976.

203. **Wallace, S. M., Runikis, J. O., and Stewart, W. D.,** The effect of pH on *in-vitro* percutaneous penetration of methotrexate: correlation with solubility and partition coefficient, *Can. J. Pharm. Sci.*, 13, 66, 1978.

204. **Cohen, J. L. and Stoughton, R. B.,** Penetration of 5-fluorouracil in excised skin, *J. Invest. Dermatol.*, 62, 507, 1974.

205. **Lorenzetti, O. J.,** Propylene glycol gel vehicles, *Cutis*, 23, 747, 1979.

206. **Turi, J. S., Danielson, D., and Woltersom, J. W.,** Effects of polyoxpropylene 15 stearyl ether and propylene glycol on percutaneous penetration rate of diflorasone diacetate, *J. Pharm. Sci.*, 68, 275, 1979.

207. **Dillaha, C. J., Jansen, G., Honeycutt, W. M., and Holt, C. A.,** Further studies with topical 5-fluorouracil, *Arch. Dermatol.*, 92, 410, 1965.

208. **Molgaard, B., Hoelgaard, A., and Bundgaard, H.,** Prodrugs as drug delivery systems. XXIII. Improved dermal delivery of 5-fluorouracil through human skin via *N*-acyloxymethyl prodrug derivatives, *Int. J. Pharm.*, 12, 153, 1982.

209. **Yu, C. D., Higuchi, W., Ho, N., Fox, J., and Flynn, G.,** Physical model evaluation of topical prodrug delivery — simultaneous transport and bioconversion of vidarabine-5'-valerate. III. Permeability differences of vidarabine and *n*-pentanol in components of hairless mouse skin, *J. Pharm. Sci.*, 69, 770, 1980.

210. **Spruance, S. L., McKeough, M. B., and Cardinal, J. R.,** Dimethyl sulfoxide as a vehicle for topical antiviral chemotherapy, *Ann. N. Y. Acad. Sci.*, 411, 28, 1983.

211. **Sloan, K. B., Hashida, M., Alexander, J., Bodor, N., and Higuchi, T.,** Prodrugs of 6-thiopurines: enhanced delivery through the skin, *J. Pharm. Sci.*, 72, 372, 1983.

212. **Bailey, D. N. and Briggs, J. R.,** Ethanol inhibition of phencyclidine percutaneous absorption, *Life Sci.*, 34, 757, 1984.

Index

INDEX